COLOUR GUIDE

PICTURE TES

NHS Staff Library at

☎ 0113 39 ~~2644 5~~ 2014O

This book must be returned by the date shown
below or a fine will be charged.

2 4 APR 2009	3/12/20.
1 4 SEP 2009	~~2 2 JUN 2021~~
0 8 FEB 2010	1 2 MAY 2021
1 2 AUG 2010	
- 6 MAY 2011	
2 5 MAY 2011	

EDINBURGH LONDON NEW YORK PHILADELPHIA ST LOUIS SYDNEY TORONTO
1999

CHURCHILL LIVINGSTONE
An imprint of Harcourt Publishers Limited

First published 1999

ISBN 0443 06235 8

British Library Cataloguing in Publication Data
A catalogue record for this book is available from the British
Library

Library of Congress Cataloging in Publication Data
A catalog record for this book is available from the Library of
Congress

Note
Medical knowledge is constantly changing. As new
information becomes available, changes in treatment,
procedures, equipment and the use of drugs become
necessary. The authors and the publishers have, as far as it is
possible, taken care to ensure that the information given in
this text is accurate and up-to-date. However, readers are
strongly advised to confirm that the information, expecially
with regard to drug usage, complies with the latest legislation
and standards of practice.

Commissioning Editor
Michael Parkinson

Project Editor
Jim Killgore

Project Controller
Frances Affleck

Designer
Erik Bigland

Printed in China
SWTC/01

Preface

ENT surgery is a specialty that manages conditions of the head and neck, with the exception of those that affect the eye. It is perhaps now more commonly called otorhinolaryngology. Symptoms and disease are common in the head and neck, both in adults and children, hence a basic knowledge of otorhinolaryngology is required of all clinicians. In the United Kingdom, the majority of such conditions are managed by primary care physicians (general practitioners). It is important for them to be able to examine the ear, nose, mouth, oropharynx, neck and to test the hearing in order to identify pathology. They also have to recognise when onward referral to an otorhinolaryngologist for investigation and management is required.

This text attempts to educate the non-specialist in these tasks, many of the photographs being used to introduce a topic rather than as a spot diagnosis. Conditions of the ear, particularly those of the external auditory canal, middle ear and inner ear, require special techniques including otoscopy and audiology that are not applicable to any other region. Hence this text is divided into two sections—Otology and Audiology, and General Otorhinolaryngology.

G.W. McG.
G.G.B.

Preface to Otology and Audiology Section

The otoscopic photographs in this text come from *Otoscopy—A Structured Approach* by P.J. Wormald and G.G. Browning, published by Arnold, London, 1996 (ISBN 0 340 613769). The publishers and Mr. P.J. Wormald are thanked for permission to use them. In the Suggested Reading on page 132 each photograph is referenced by its figure number in *Otoscopy—A Structured Approach* so that further reading of this text as to how to arrive at a diagnosis and manage a patient is made easy.

G.G.B.

Preface to General Otorhinolaryngology Section

In putting together the general otolaryngology section, I have tried to avoid inclusion of bizarre or unusual conditions. Therefore, most of the conditions covered are commonly encountered in everyday otorhinolaryngological practice. The selection of slides has come almost exclusively from my own collection and I have first-hand knowledge of most of the cases described. The explanations of the questions are fairly detailed and, where repetition occurs, it is deliberate and intended to reinforce an important clinical message. Ideally, a 'first-pass' attempt at the question should be made and then an appropriate textbook from the reading list consulted. Following this background reading, the questions should then be attempted seriously aiming to answer each of the stems in as much detail as possible.

I would like to acknowledge the assistance of Mr. Kenneth MacKenzie and Mr. Iain R.C. Swan, who have allowed me to take a few slides from their personal collections. I would also like to thank the surgical trainees who assisted me in identifying suitable cases for photographing. Grant Robertson deserves special mention for this.

G.W. McG.

Contents

Otology and Audiology—
    questions   1
General
    Otorhinolaryngology—
    questions   39
Otology and Audiology—
    answers   102
General
    Otorhinolaryngology—
    answers   112
Suggested reading   132

Index   133

Otology and Audiology— Questions

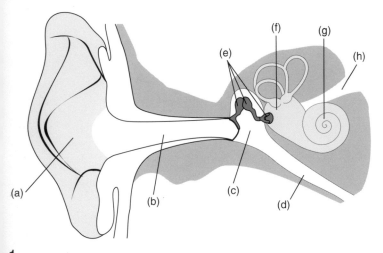

1. Name the lettered parts of this drawing of a coronal section of the ear.

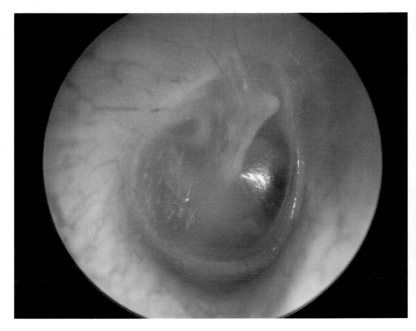

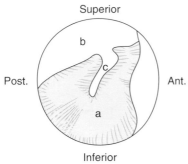

Superior

Post.　　　　　　Ant.

Inferior

2. **This is a photograph of the right tympanic membrane. Name the parts marked alphabetically.**

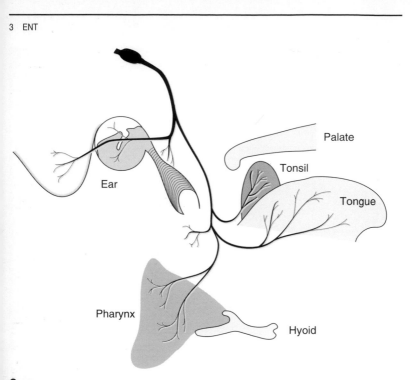

3. **This is a diagram of the sensory distribution of one of the cranial nerves.**

a. Which cranial nerve is it?
b. Why is this nerve relevant in some patients with otalgia (pain in the ear)?

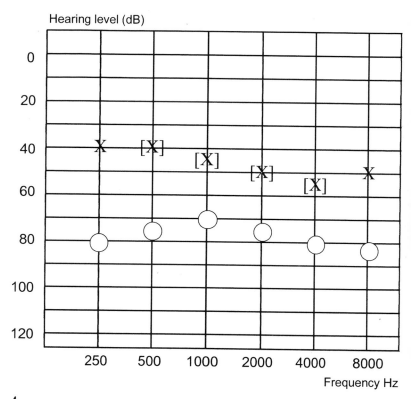

Hearing level (dB) / Frequency Hz

4. This is a patient's pure-tone audiogram:

a. How is pure-tone audiometry carried out?
b. What can it show?
c. What does it show in this particular patient?

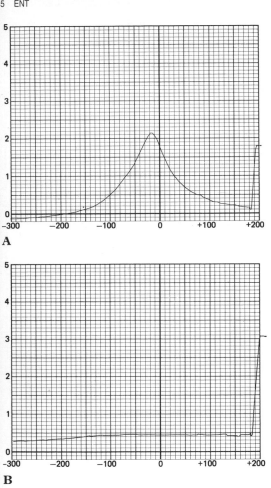

A

B

5. The first photograph (A) is of a normal tympanogram. The second photograph (B) is of a tympanogram from an ear in a child aged 3 years with a suspected hearing impairment. What is the likely diagnosis that can be made from the second tympanogram?

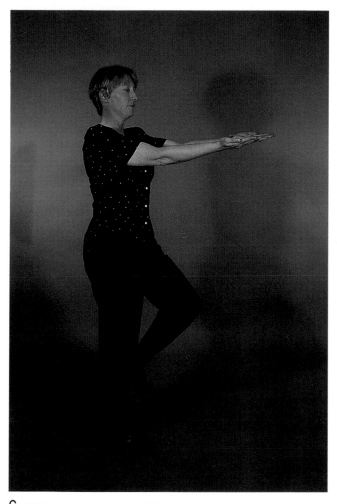

6. **This patient is marching on the spot, with her eyes closed and her arms outstretched with the palms upwards in the Unterberger test.**

a. What is being tested in this test?
b. What would happen if there was an abnormality?

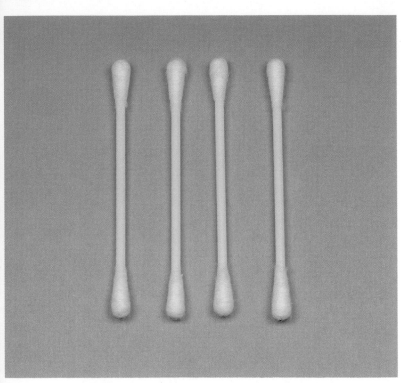

7. How often should a normal ear be cleaned with these to remove wax?

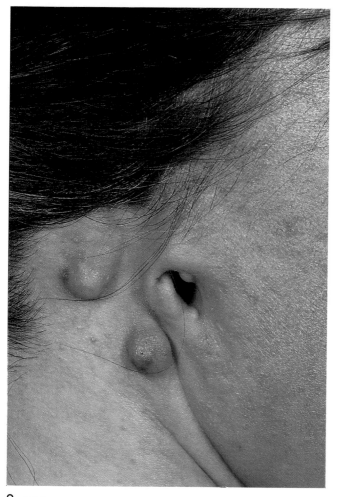

8. This child has been born with a congenital abnormality affecting both ears.

a. What should be the main concern in such a child?
b. How is this managed?
c. Is this the commonest type of congenital ear pathology?

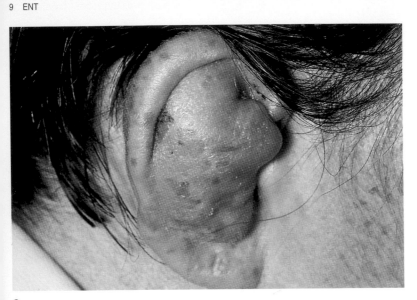

9. This young lad was playing rugby and injured his right ear in a scrum.

a. What is the diagnosis?
b. What requires to be done?
c. What is the likely outcome if this condition is not managed correctly?

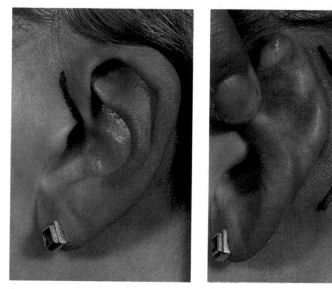

A   B

10. These photographs are inked lines illustrating the sites of the two commonest surgical skin incisions for ear surgery. What is each called and what type of surgery is likely to have been carried out through each of them?

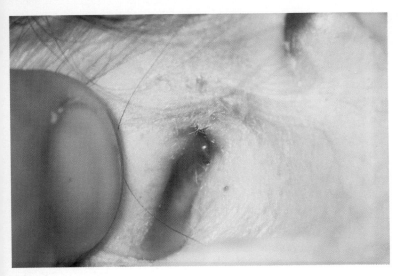

11. This adult patient has a discharging right ear.

a. What are the two most likely causes?
b. How is the cause ascertained?

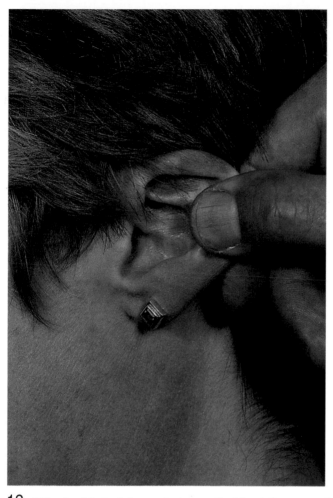

12. Why is this lady's ear being pulled in this manner?

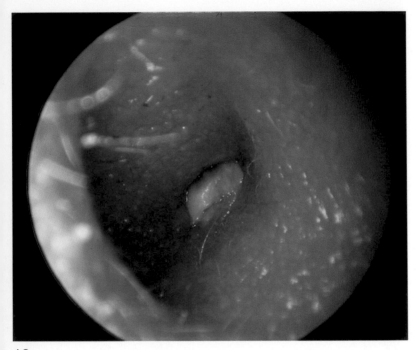

13. This patient has an acutely painful, tender left ear. Otoscopy is uncomfortable and this is all that can be seen of the external auditory canal.

a. What is the diagnosis?
b. What is the management?

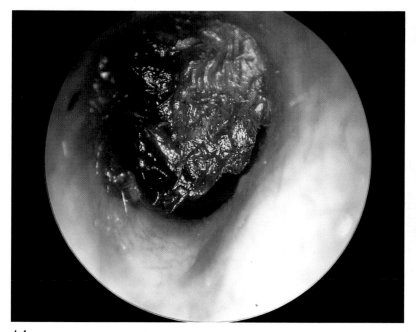

14. **This is the right ear of a patient complaining of a hearing impairment.**

a. What is seen otoscopically?
b. What requires to be done?
c. Is this likely to be the cause of the hearing impairment?

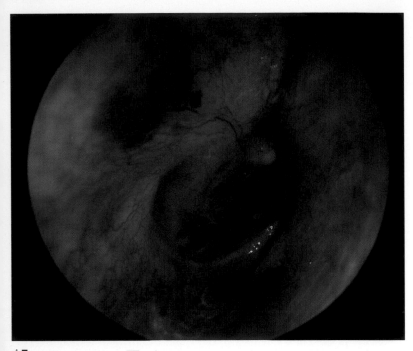

15. This right ear has recently been syringed to remove wax.

a. What can be seen?
b. What are the complications of syringing?

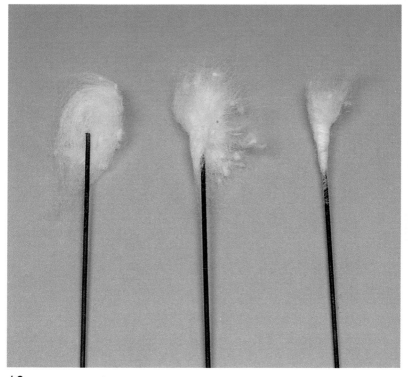

16. This photograph illustrates how to make a fine cotton bud that is used in the management of some otological conditions. What are these conditions?

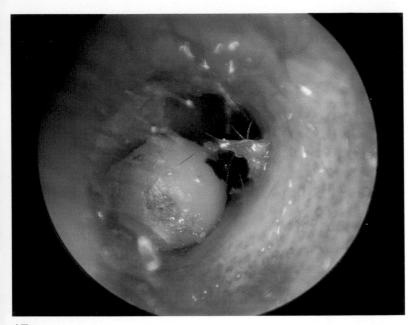

17. A young boy is brought by his mother who says he has been rubbing his right ear for the last few days, presumably because it is sore.

a. What can be seen on the photograph of his external auditory canal?
b. What should be done about it?
c. How could this have occurred and why?

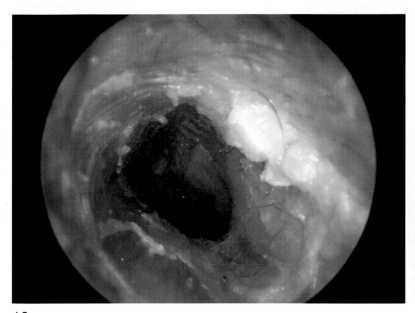

18. This patient has recently been on holiday in the Mediterranean and has an uncomfortable, itchy, slightly discharging left ear.

a. What is the diagnosis?

b. What is the management?

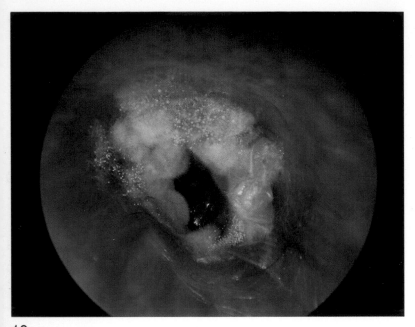

19. This patient has had a course of topical antibiotic steroid ear drops for otitis externa.

a. What complication has occurred?
b. What other complications are there of such drops?

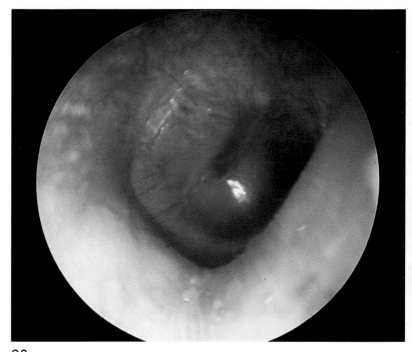

20. This is the right tympanic membrane in a crying, 18-month-old child with an upper respiratory infection, fever and perhaps otalgia.

a. What is the differential diagnosis?
b. How should this child be managed?

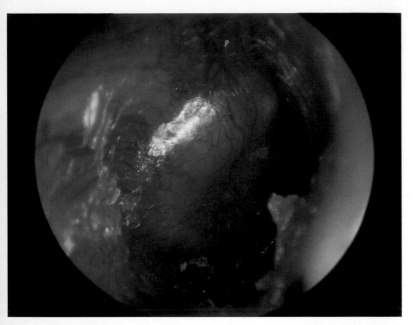

21. This is the right tympanic membrane in a one-year-old child with fever and otalgia.

a. What is the diagnosis?
b. What is the management of this child in the first 24–48 hours?
c. What is the management thereafter?

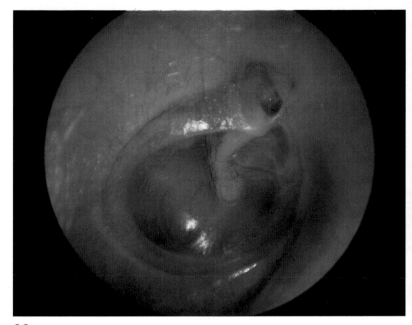

22. This is the right ear in a 4-year-old girl whose parents are concerned about her hearing. The other ear is similar in appearance.

a. What is the diagnosis?
b. What investigations could be done?
c. How should this child be managed in the first instance?

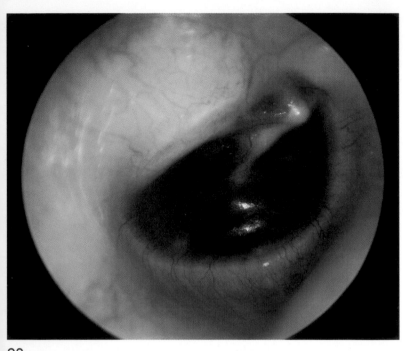

23. This is the otoscopic appearance of the right ear in a 2-year-old boy with recurrent episodes of otalgia, though not at the present time. The other ear appears the same.

a. What is the diagnosis?
b. What should be done?

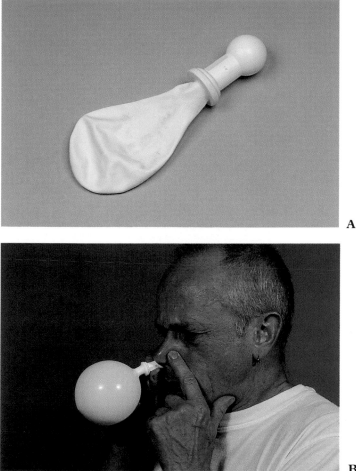

A

B

24.

a. What is this patient doing?
b. Why might he be doing this?
c. Is this technique applicable in children?
d. What is the technique called if performed without a balloon?

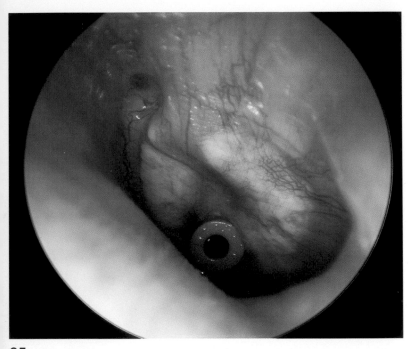

25. This 4-year-old child has recently had an operation on both ears to improve the hearing which was impaired due to otitis media with effusion. This is a photograph of the left tympanic membrane post-operatively.

a. What operation has been performed?
b. How does this work?
c. What is likely to happen in about 6 months time?

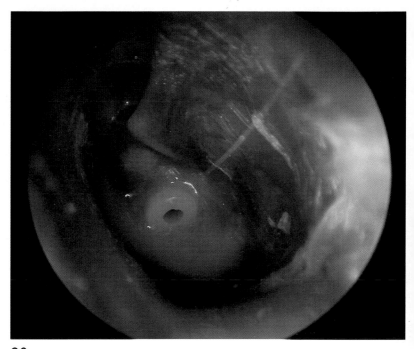

26. **This 4-year-old boy has developed a foul smelling left ear discharge after a recent operation.**

a. What operation has been carried out?
b. What complication has occurred?
c. How is this managed?
d. What may be the end result?

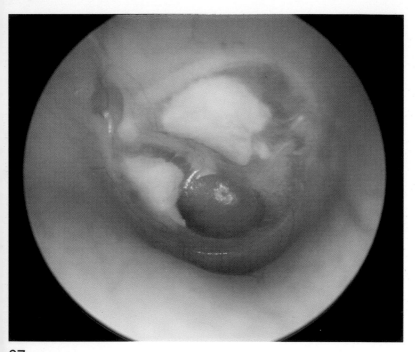

27. **This is the left ear of a 29-year-old man with no ear symptoms. The other ear is similar in appearance.**

a. What are the otoscopic findings?
b. What are the predisposing conditions for these findings?
c. What is the natural history of this condition?

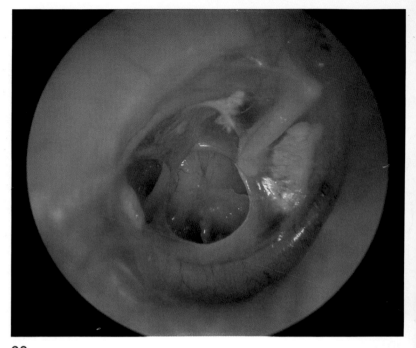

28. This 35-year-old patient complains of a hearing impairment in his right ear.

a. What is the otoscopic diagnosis?
b. What are the alternative methods of alleviating his hearing impairment?

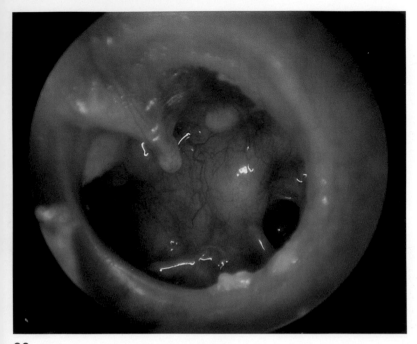

29. This 29-year-old female complains of a hearing impairment in her left ear with an occasional ear discharge that is foul smelling.

a. What is the diagnosis?
b. What is the management?

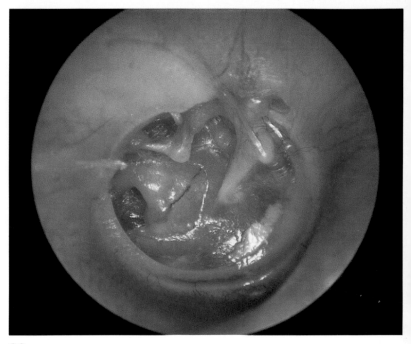

30. This is the right ear of a 19-year-old lad who has a hearing impairment and a long history of trouble with his ears as a child.

a. What is seen otoscopically?
b. What condition is he likely to have had as a child?
c. What is the management?

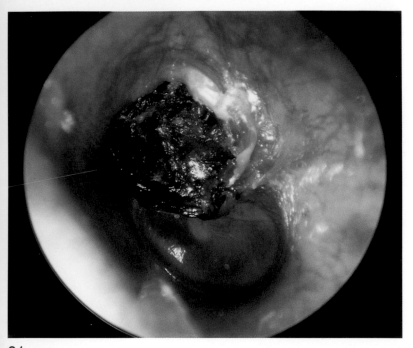

31. **This is the left ear of a patient who complains of imbalance of recent onset.**

a. What can be seen?
b. What should be done?

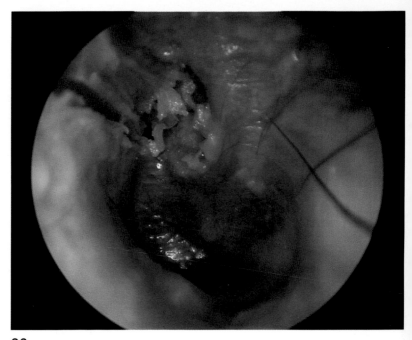

32. This is the left ear, after cleaning out of debris, in a patient who complains of imbalance.

a. What can be seen?
b. Why does the patient experience imbalance?
c. What requires to be done?

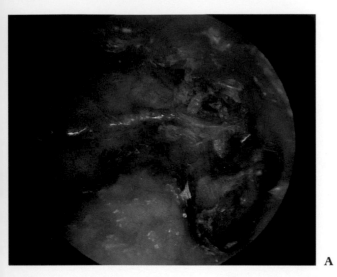

A

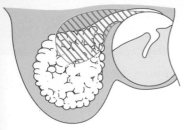

B

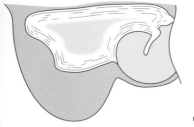

C

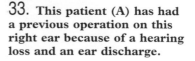

33. This patient (A) has had a previous operation on this right ear because of a hearing loss and an ear discharge.

a. What operation (B & C) has the patient had?

b. What condition would they have had the operation for?

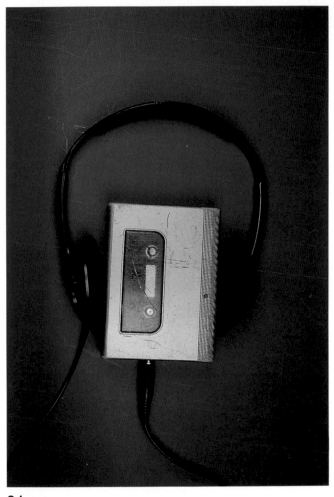

34. This is a personal stereo.

a. What health warning should come with it?
b. What other hobbies or social activities should be so labelled?

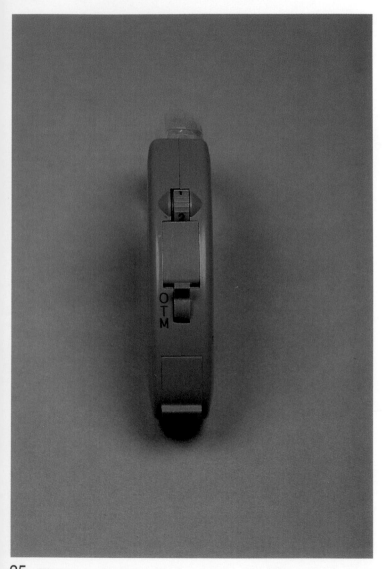

35. These are the controls the patient can adjust on a behind-the-ear aid. What do they do?

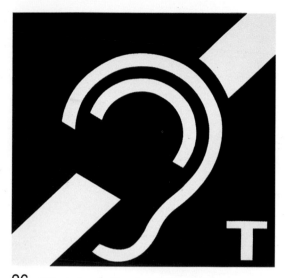

36. What does this sign indicate?

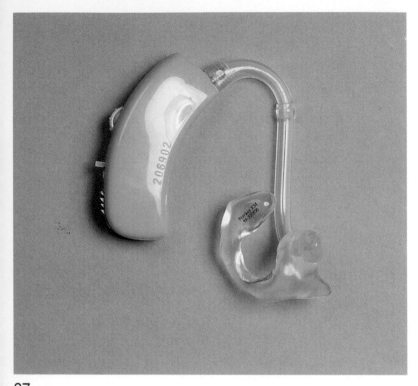

37. This looks like a hearing aid but it only produces a 'noise'. What is it and what symptom is it used to alleviate?

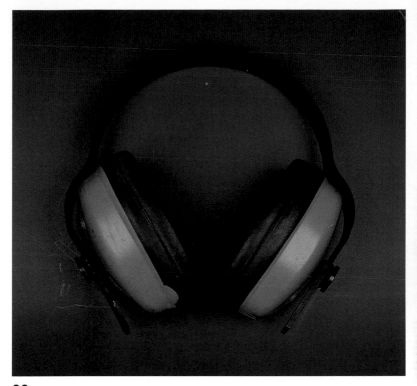

38. **When should these be worn?**

General Otorhinolaryngology —Questions

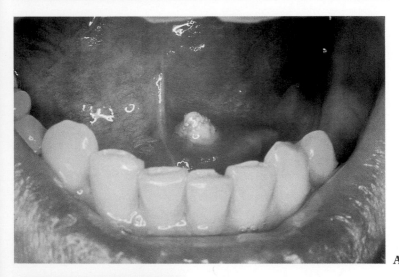

A

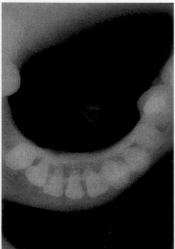

B

39. A 37-year-old male presented with a 3-month history of intermittent swelling beneath his left lower jaw, associated with pain and discomfort when eating. Picture A is an intraoral view and picture B is a plain radiograph of the anterior floor of mouth.

a. What is shown in picture A and confirmed on the radiograph in picture B?
b. How is this condition managed?
c. Why is the lesion commoner in this site?
d. What are the possible complications of this condition?

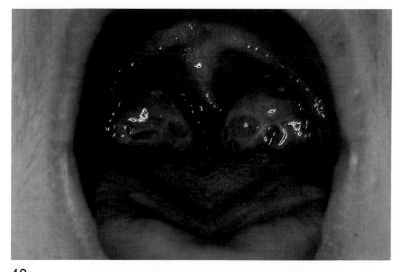

40. This 16-year-old male developed an acute sore throat which was treated with antibiotics on the advice of his general practitioner. The pain failed to settle and he was referred to an otorhinolaryngologist 4 weeks after the onset of his symptoms. In addition to sore throat, he complained of generalised malaise and enlargement of his cervical glands. He had lost his appetite and his parents noticed that he had started to snore!

a. Describe the clinical features on oropharyngeal examination.
b. What investigations would you carry out on this patient?
c. What is the most likely diagnosis?
d. Why is the patient snoring at night?

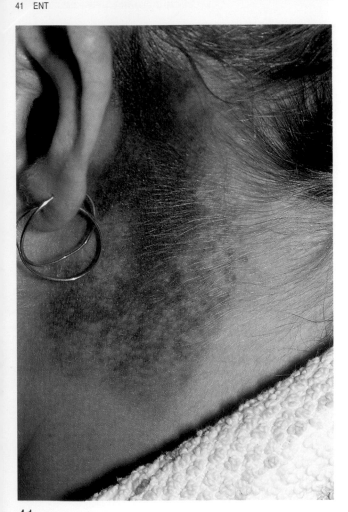

41. This 60-year-old woman tripped over a rug and struck the left side of her head against a tiled floor. She was unconscious for a few minutes and, on regaining consciousness, she felt dizzy and had ringing in her left ear. She was so severely dizzy that she was unable to walk without assistance.

a. What does the picture show and what is the name of this clinical sign?
b. What is the most likely diagnosis?
c. Why is the patient unable to walk without assistance?
d. What investigations would you request on such a patient?

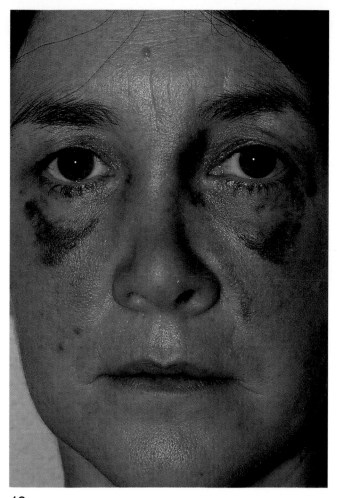

42. **This patient sustained facial injuries in an assault. She complained of bilateral nasal obstruction and numbness in the region of her left cheek.**

a. List the abnormalities shown in the picture.
b. Why might she be suffering from nasal obstruction?
c. What is the cause of the numbness in her left cheek?
d. How would you manage her nasal injury?

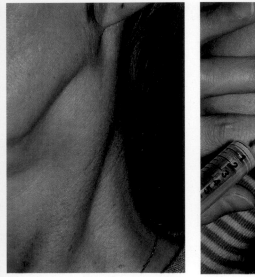
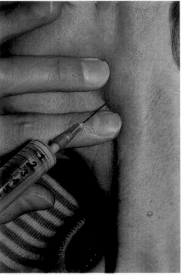

A **B**

43. A 30-year-old woman presented to the clinic with a 2-month history of a slowly enlarging swelling in the left upper neck. The lesion is shown in photograph A and is being investigated in photograph B.

a. What is the differential diagnosis of a neck lump in this position?
b. What investigation is being performed in photograph B?
c. Look closely at photograph B and use all the available information to suggest the most likely diagnosis?
d. What examinations must be carried out on patients with neck swellings?

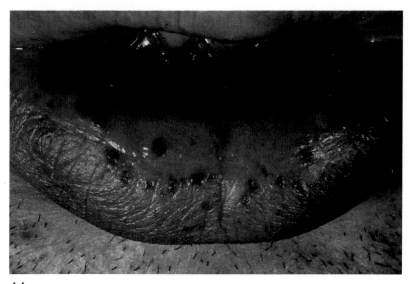

44. This 25-year-old male presented with recurrent epistaxis. Investigation revealed an iron deficiency anaemia.

a. What are the lesions shown in the photograph?
b. What condition is this patient suffering from? What is its mode of transmission and what is its eponymous title?
c. What is the most likely cause of his iron deficiency anaemia?
d. What treatment options are available for his troublesome epistaxis?

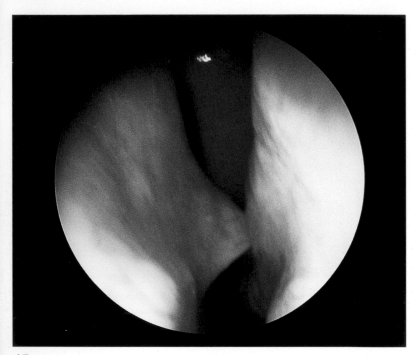

45. This patient presented with left-sided nasal obstruction. Examination of the left nasal cavity revealed the features shown in the picture.

a. What abnormality is demonstrated in the picture?
b. What is the cause of such an abnormality?
c. How is the abnormality treated?

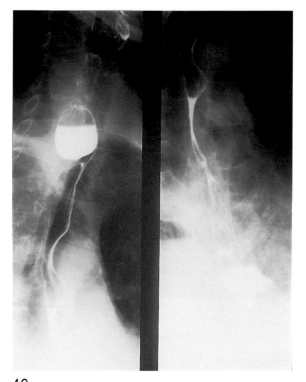

46. An 80-year-old male presented with a 2-year history of gradually worsening dysphagia. He described food sticking in his throat and episodes of regurgitation of undigested foodstuffs. He had been otherwise fit and well but had been admitted to hospital with an episode of pneumonia 6 months prior to his attendance in the Otorhinolaryngology Clinic. Examination was essentially negative but the findings of the radiological investigation are shown in the photograph.

a. What investigation is this and what does it show?
b. How does such a lesion cause dysphagia?
c. What is the possible relationship between this lesion and the patient's recent admission to hospital with pneumonia?
d. What treatment options are available for this lesion?

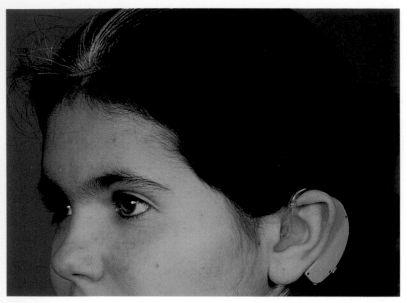

47.

a. Describe the features shown in the photograph.
b. What is the diagnosis?
c. What is its mode of transmission?

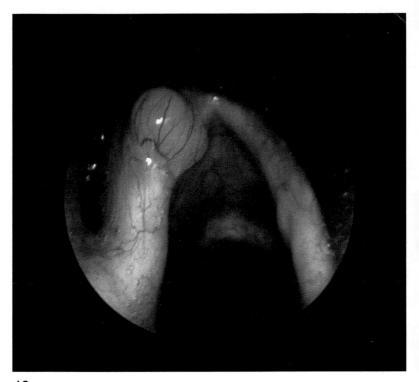

48. This endolaryngeal photograph shows a lesion on the anterior end of the left true vocal cord.

a. What symptom would this patient complain of?
b. What is the differential diagnosis of this symptom?
c. How might this lesion be treated?

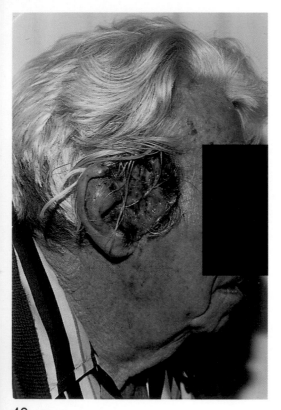

49. This patient worked on a sheep farm in the Australian outback.

a. What does the picture show?
b. What is the differential diagnosis?
c. What is the relevance of the geographic information in the history?
d. What are the treatment options available?

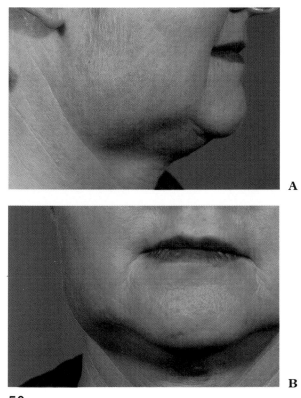

A

B

50. This patient presented with a slowly enlarging right facial swelling, as shown in photographs A and B.

a. What is the differential diagnosis of a swelling in this region?

b. What investigations would help you reach a diagnosis?

c. When is incisional biopsy recommended?

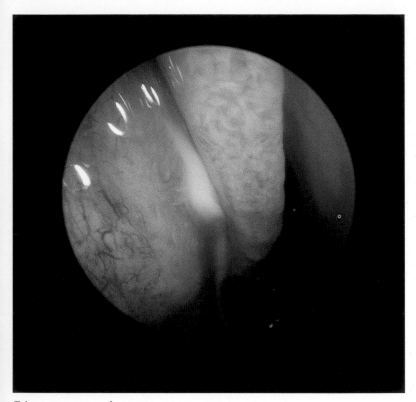

51. A 28-year-old male presented with a 3-week history of nasal congestion, right facial pain, headache, fever and purulent nasal discharge. The photograph is an endoscopic view of the right nasal cavity centred on the right middle nasal meatus.

a. Describe the abnormalities shown in the photograph.
b. What is the diagnosis?
c. How would you investigate and manage this patient?

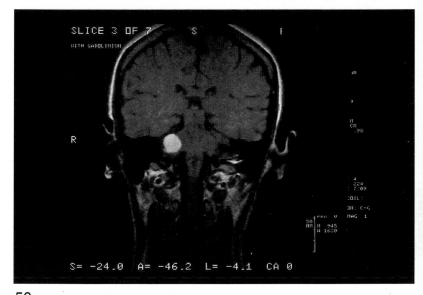

SLICE 3 OF 7   S   I

WITH GADOLINIUM

R

S= -24.0   A= -46.2   L= -4.1   CA 0

52. This patient presented with decreased hearing and unilateral right tinnitus. There were no symptoms from the left ear.

a. What investigation is shown?
b. What is the diagnosis?
c. What is the first line investigation for such a patient?

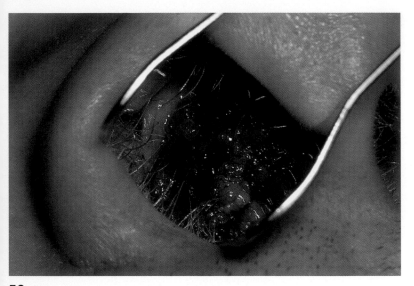

53. **This 35-year-old male presented with a 6-month history of bleeding and discharge from the right nostril.**

a. Describe the features shown in the photograph.
b. What is the differential diagnosis?
c. What is the causal agent in this condition?

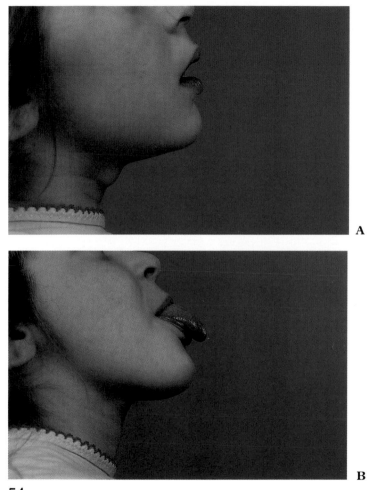

A

B

54. This 10-year-old girl presented with the slowly enlarging painless neck swelling shown in photograph A.

a. What is the differential diagnosis of this neck lump?
b. Describe what is occurring in photograph B.
c. What does the treatment of this lesion involve?

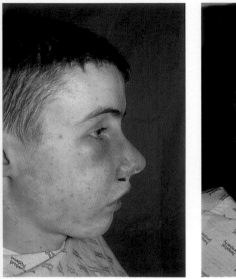
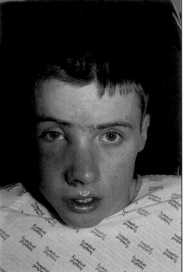

A   **B**

55. Photographs A and B show the clinical appearance in a
14-year-old male who presented with a 1-week history of fever,
right facial pain, headache, nasal obstruction and rhinorrhoea.

a. Describe the clinical features.
b. What is the most likely diagnosis and its cause?
c. How should this case be managed?
d. Name two other complications of this condition.

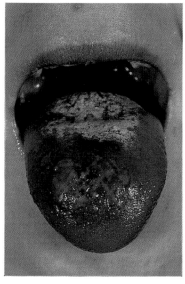 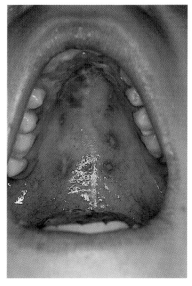

A   **B**

56. A 14-year-old girl presented to the clinic with a 1-week history of painful mouth ulcers, painful tongue and general malaise. The pain was so severe that she was unable to eat or drink and had become dehydrated.

a. Describe the features shown on photographs A and B.
b. What is the differential diagnosis?
c. How would you confirm the diagnosis?
d. List the steps in management of this patient.

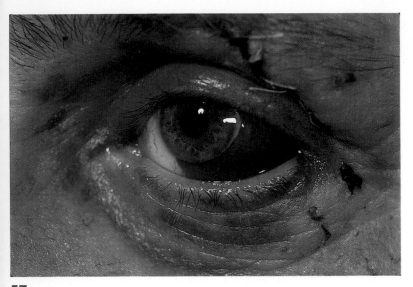

57. This elderly male was involved in a road traffic accident. His face and forehead struck the steering wheel.

a. What is the clinical sign shown in the photograph and what are the two main categories of this sign?
b. What are the implications of this finding for the patient?
c. This patient also complained of unilateral watery rhinorrhoea. How would you decide whether this was CSF rhinorrhoea or not?

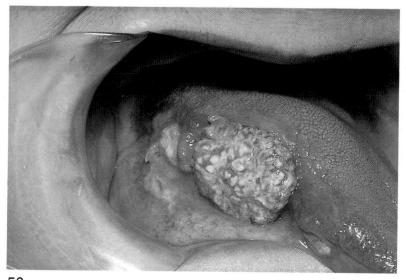

58. **A 60-year-old male smoker presented to the clinic with a painless, slowly enlarging lesion on the lateral border of his tongue.**

a. What is the most likely diagnosis?
b. How would you establish a diagnosis in this case?
c. What other regions of the head and neck would you examine and why?

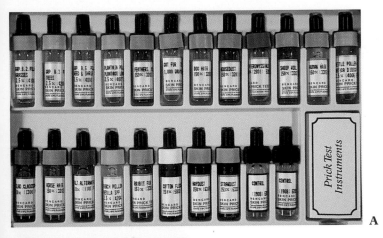

A

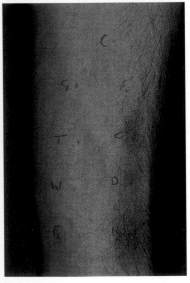

B

59. Photographs A and B show the reagents and results of a test commonly carried out at rhinology clinics.

a. What is the test? How and why is it employed at a rhinology clinic?

b. During such a test, the patient suddenly collapsed, became breathless and had no detectable pulse. What has occurred and how will you manage the emergency?

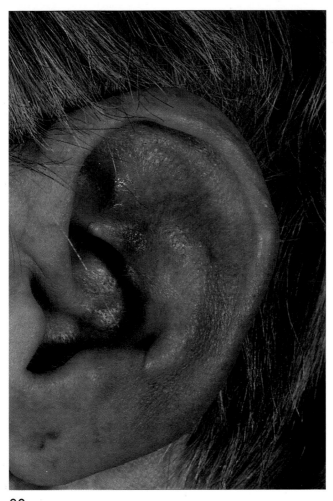

60. This patient presented with a 3-month history of a non-healing lesion on the left pinna.

a. What is the differential diagnosis?
b. How would you establish a diagnosis?
c. What are the treatment options?
d. Which other parts of the head and neck would you examine in this patient?

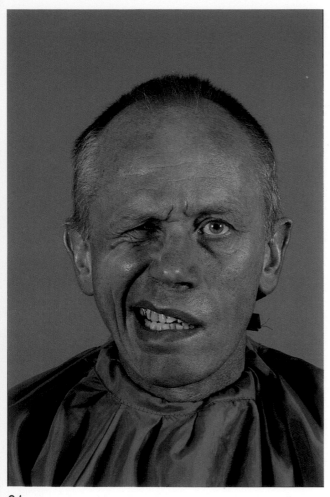

61. The clinical findings in this 53-year-old academic ENT surgeon are shown in the photograph.

a. What is the diagnosis and which is the affected side?
b. Give four possible causes of this condition.
c. Assuming this is of idiopathic origin, how would you manage the condition?

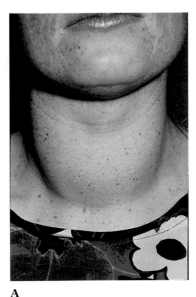

A

62. A 44-year-old woman presented to the clinic with gradually enlarging swelling of her neck (A). She had also noticed that she was becoming dysphonic (hoarse). Photograph B is an axial MRI scan of her neck at the level of C6.

a. Describe the features shown in both photographs and suggest a diagnosis.
b. How might a definitive diagnosis be established?
c. Why might the patient be dysphonic?

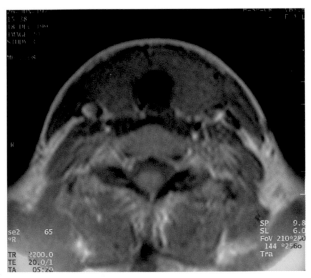

B

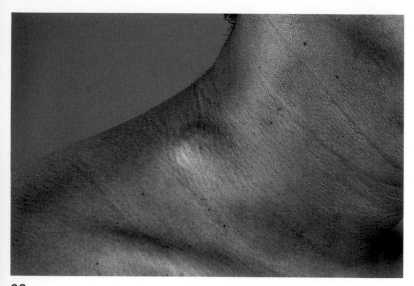

63. An 18-year-old patient presented to the clinic with the painless swelling shown in the photograph. There was no other abnormality on examination of the head and neck.

a. Describe the lesion, in particular, noting its position in the neck.
b. What is the differential diagnosis?
c. How would the diagnosis be established in this case?
d. If excision of this node is considered, what structure is at particular risk?

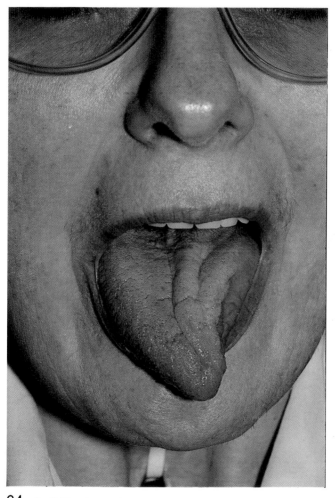

64. A difficult one! Look closely and take account of all of the information in the photograph.

a. What clinical sign is shown here?
b. What is the most likely cause in this patient? (Look closely at the photograph.)

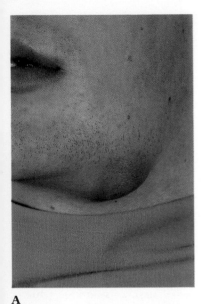

65. This 22-year-old man presented with a 4-day history of increasing pain in the left lower jaw and swelling of the upper neck on the left. He was systemically unwell with a high fever and raised white blood cell count.

a. Describe photographs A and B and make a diagnosis.
b. How should this condition be treated?
c. What is the most likely organism involved? How does it affect your choice of antibiotics?

A

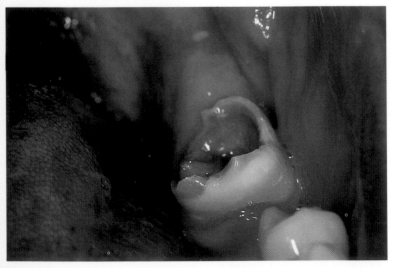

B

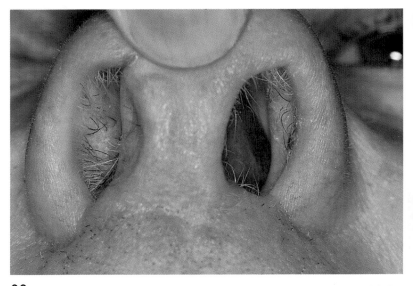

66. This patient presented with bilateral nasal obstruction which was worse on the left. The photograph shows the findings on anterior rhinoscopy. Look closely at the photograph, pay attention to the abnormality visible in each of the nostrils and answer the following questions.

a. What is the abnormality in the right nostril and how does it relate to the abnormality in the left nostril?
b. What is the diagnosis?
c. What is the aetiology of this condition?
d. What is the treatment?

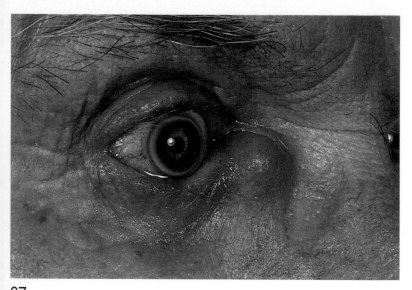

67. **This 70-year-old male gives a history of recurrent inflammation in the region of the medial canthus of the right eye.**

a. What two, unrelated, abnormalities are shown?
b. What is the most likely diagnosis?
c. What has this got to do with otolaryngology? (Think about how you would treat it.)

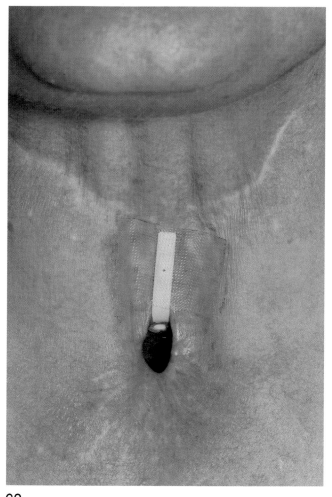

68. Study the photograph. List the abnormalities and answer the following questions.

a. What operation has this patient had and what was the most likely diagnosis?

b. What is the white structure visible in the photograph and what is its purpose?

c. What are the alternatives to such a prosthesis?

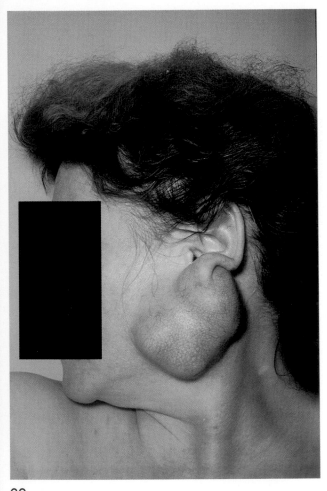

69. This patient presented with a 6-year history of a slowly enlarging lesion as shown in the photograph.

a. What is the most likely diagnosis?
b. How would this diagnosis be confirmed?
c. How is this condition treated?

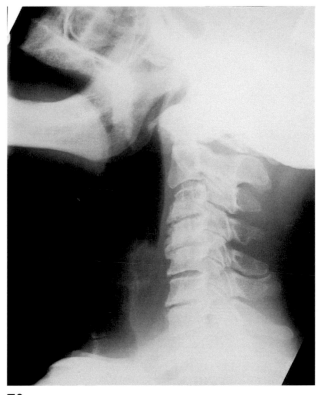

70. **This 80-year-old female presented with increasing difficulty swallowing solids. The photograph shows the findings on lateral soft tissue X-ray.**

a. Describe the radiological findings?
b. What is the most likely diagnosis?
c. How would this patient be investigated?
d. What are the treatment options in this patient?

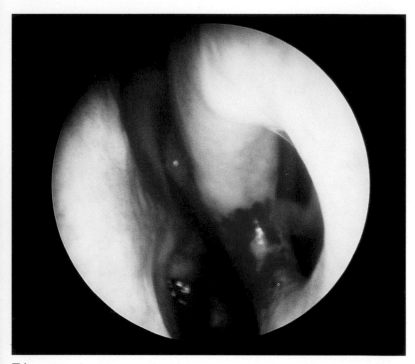

71. This patient complained of intermittent nasal bleeding and a whistling noise when breathing through his nose! The photograph shows the clinical appearance on examination of his right nostril.

a. What does the photograph show?
b. Give *five* causes of this condition?
c. How can this condition be managed?

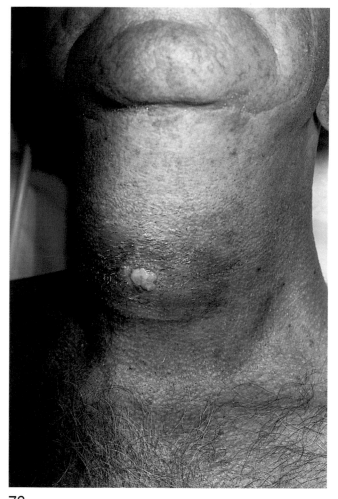

72. This 57-year-old heavy smoker presented with a history of noisy breathing, breathlessness and difficulty in swallowing. The photograph shows the appearance on examination of his neck.

a. Describe the features shown?
b. What is the most likely diagnosis?
c. How would this patient be managed?

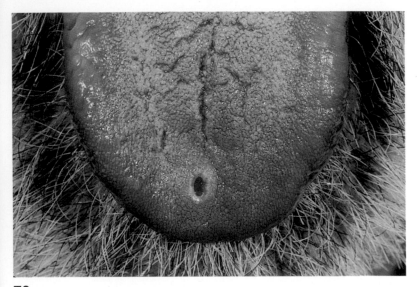

73. This bearded gentleman presented with a 6-week history of a lesion on the tip of his tongue.

a. What is the differential diagnosis of this ulcer?
b. List the steps in assessment of this patient.
c. To which side of the neck do the lymphatics of this part of the tongue drain?

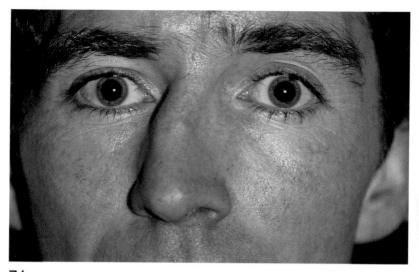

74. This patient presented to the clinic complaining of nasal obstruction and a deformed nose following a nasal injury some 10 years prior to the consultation.

a. Describe the nasal abnormalities shown in the picture.
b. From these abnormalities, can you deduce the most likely mechanism of trauma?
c. What procedure is used to correct these deformities?

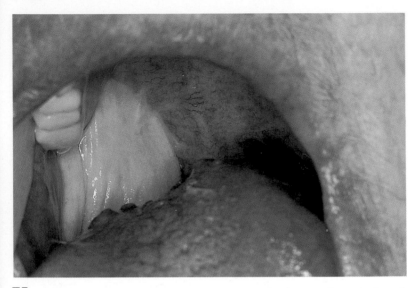

75. This is an intraoral view of a patient who has undergone head and neck surgery for carcinoma.

a. From the information on the photograph, what procedure do you think the patient has undergone?
b. List problem areas in the rehabilitation of such patients.
c. Some authorities recommend that patients who have this condition should have annual chest X-rays. Why?

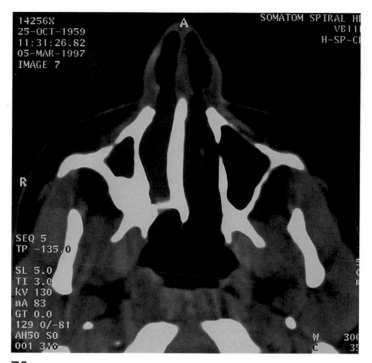

76. This is an axial CT scan at the level of the nose and nasopharynx in a young adult who presented with unilateral nasal obstruction.

a. What and where is the abnormality?
b. When is this condition usually diagnosed?
c. How can this condition be managed?

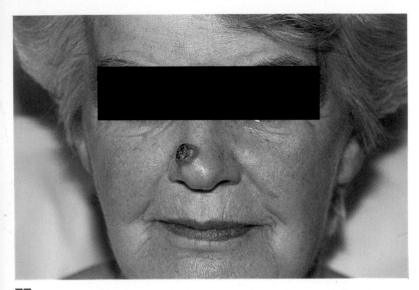

77. This patient presented with a rapidly enlarging disfiguring lesion on the tip of her nose.

a. List the differential diagnosis.
b. How might this lesion be treated?
c. If surgery is used, how is the defect reconstructed?

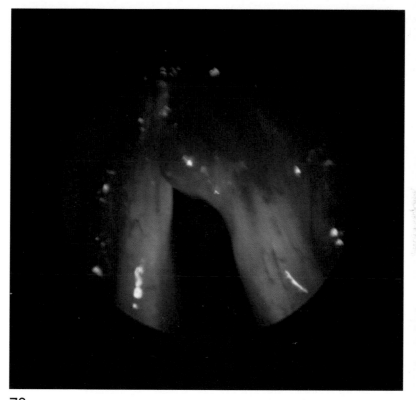

78. This 35-year-old football fan suffered severe dysphonia (hoarseness) following a football match during which he felt it necessary to shout non-constructive criticisms to the referee from the back of the stand. The photograph shows the endoscopic findings in his larynx.

a. What is the most likely diagnosis and the mechanism of its causation?
b. How could this patient be managed?
c. What advice would you give the patient following treatment of this condition?

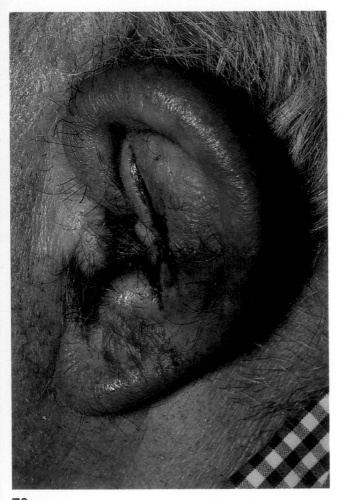

79. This patient suffered a laceration to his left pinna in an assault. He attended the Accident and Emergency Department where the wound was closed with adhesive skin closures. The photograph shows the appearance 5 days following the injury.

a. Describe the appearance of his pinna. What has occurred and what is the diagnosis?
b. How might this have been prevented?
c. How should we treat this complication?

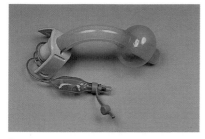

A

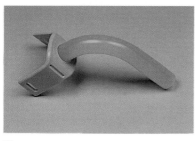

B

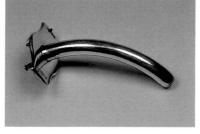

C

80. Photographs A, B and C show three different types of tracheostomy tube.

a. What is the difference between the tube in photograph A and the other two tubes? What is the function of this design difference?

b. In what circumstances might you use the tube shown in photograph B?

c. Photograph C shows a silver tracheostomy tube which is often used in long-term tracheostomies and following laryngectomy. List three important rehabilitation factors in long-term tracheostomy patients.

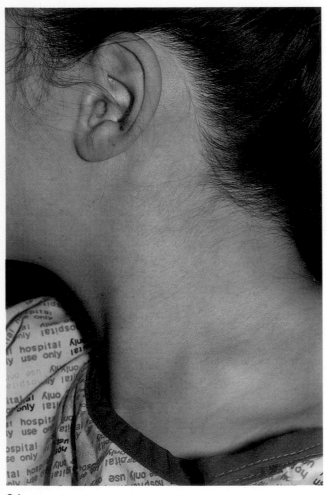

81. This patient presented with neck lumps as shown on the photograph.

a. Describe the boundaries of the anterior and posterior triangles of the neck.
b. In which triangle are these lesions situated?
c. Give three possible causes of these lumps.
d. List the steps in the investigation of this patient.

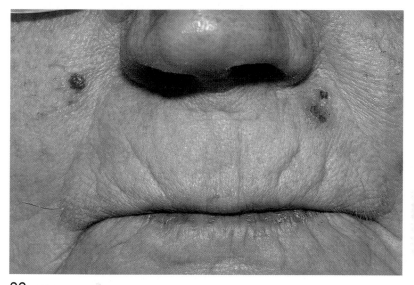

82. This patient presented with painless, persistent skin lesions shown in the photograph.

a. What is the differential diagnosis?
b. What is the management?
c. A surgical excision in this patient is likely to produce a good cosmetic result. Why?

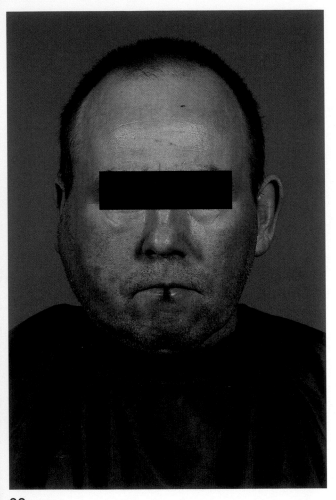

83. This patient suffered acute gastroenteritis with nausea and vomiting which lasted for several days. He then developed a high fever and the abnormalities shown in the photograph.

a. What are the two abnormalities shown in the picture?
b. What is the relevance of the history of gastroenteritis?
c. How do we treat the conditions?

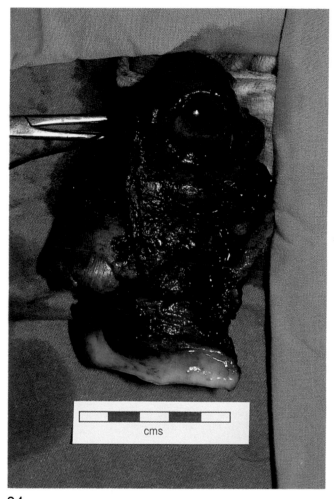

84. **This is a surgical specimen removed during a head and neck operation.**

a. What operation has been performed?
b. What is the most likely indication for this operation?
c. What are the presenting features of paranasal sinus malignancy?

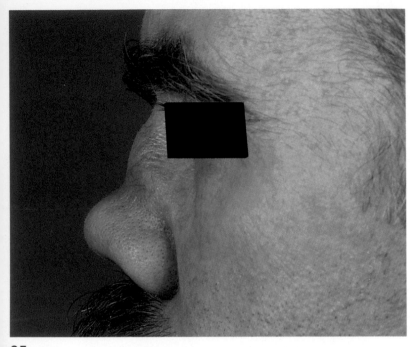

85. This patient was being treated for renal failure when his nasal deformity was brought to the attention of his local rhinologist.

a. Describe the nasal deformity.
b. List four causes of such deformity.
c. Given that this patient has been treated for renal failure, what is the possible cause in this patient?

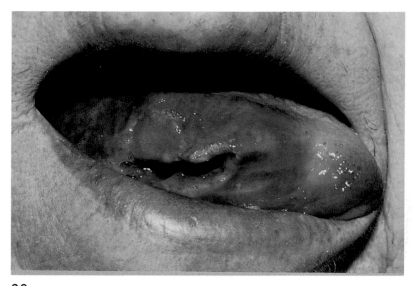

86. This 65-year-old male smoker presented with a painless lesion on the side of her tongue as shown in the photograph.

a. What is the most likely diagnosis?
b. How would this diagnosis be confirmed?
c. What other steps would be taken to investigate this patient?
d. What are the treatment options?

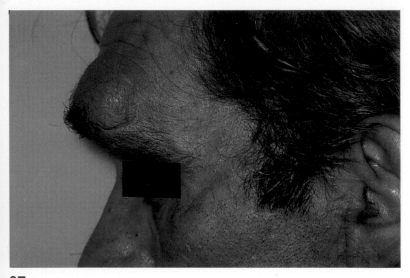

87. This patient presented with a painless, slowly enlarging lesion above his left eye.

a. What is the likely diagnosis?
b. How should this patient be investigated?
c. How might this area be approached surgically?

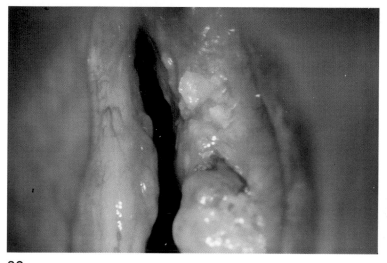

88. This is an endoscopic view of the larynx of a 57-year-old male smoker.

a. Describe the abnormality and which side is affected?
b. What is the most likely presenting symptom in this patient?
c. What is the likely diagnosis and how is it treated?

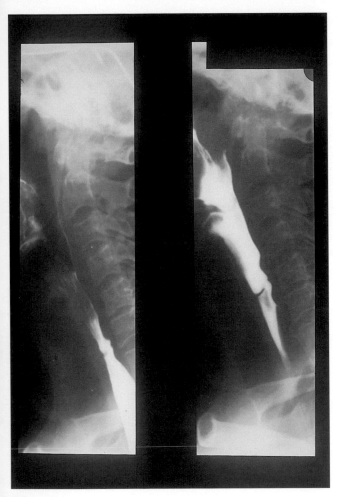

89. This is a contrast swallow radiograph from an 86-year-old female who presented with a feeling of food sticking in her throat. The patient was also found to have an iron deficiency anaemia.

a. Describe the abnormality.
b. Whose syndrome is this?
c. What is the prognosis in this condition?

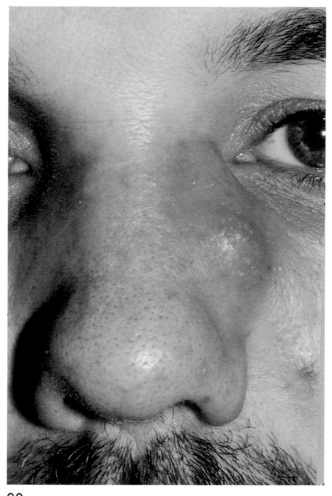

90. This young man presented to the clinic with a slowly enlarging painful, hot, red lesion to the left of his nose.

a. What is the diagnosis?
b. Why is this a particularly dangerous location for this condition?
c. How is this patient best managed?

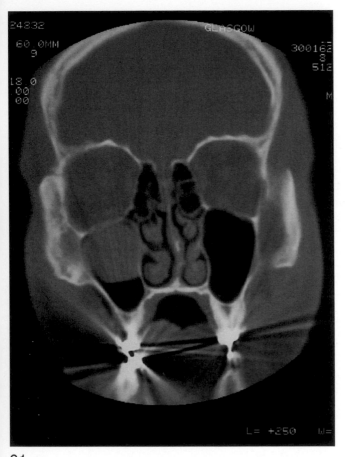

91. This patient complained of right-sided unilateral facial pain.

a. What is this investigation?
b. What and where is the abnormality?
c. How can we obtain surgical access to this region?

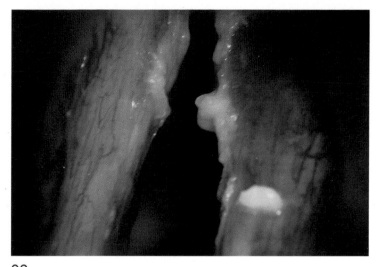

92. A 40-year-old male, heavy smoker, presented to the clinic with painless dysphonia. An endoscopic view of his vocal cords is shown in the photograph.

a. How is the larynx routinely examined in the outpatient clinic?
b. What is the descriptive term given to this appearance of the vocal cords?
c. What is the differential diagnosis?

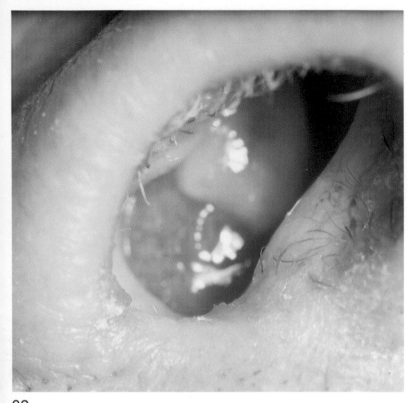

93. A 14-year-old male presented to the outpatient clinic with a 1 year history of right-sided nasal obstruction. Examination of the left nasal cavity was normal and the findings in the right nasal cavity are shown in the photograph.

a. What is the diagnosis?
b. How would you investigate this patient?
c. What is the significance of a unilateral nasal polyp?

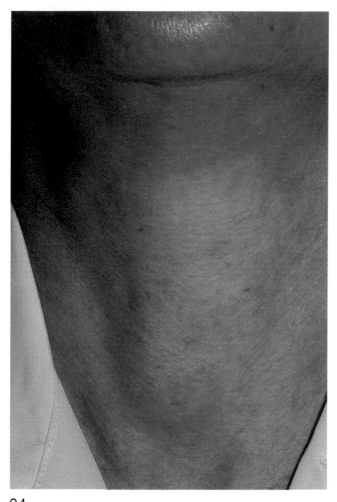

94. This 45-year-old woman presented to the clinic with a slowly enlarging lesion in her lower right neck. She also complained of dysphonia (hoarseness).

a. Describe the appearance shown in the photograph and what is the likely diagnosis?
b. How would such a neck lump be investigated?
c. What is the possible significance of her dysphonia?

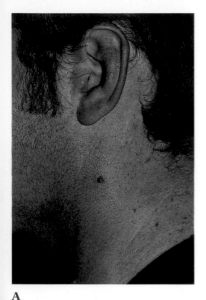

95. This patient was mowing the lawn when he suddenly felt a severe pain in the left side of his neck. He felt as if he had been struck by something. He was brought to the Accident and Emergency Department where the findings were as shown in photograph A. A lateral radiograph is shown in photograph B.

a. Look closely at the photograph and radiograph and determine what has occurred.
b. List three structures that may be damaged by penetrating neck injuries in this region.
c. List the priorities in management of this patient.

A

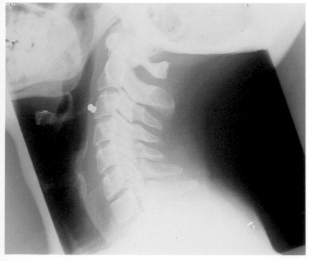

B

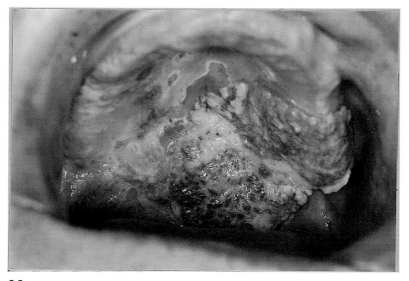

96. A 65-year-old patient presented with a painless lesion in the roof of his mouth.

a. What is the most likely diagnosis?
b. What are the aetiological factors in this condition?
c. What are the treatment options?

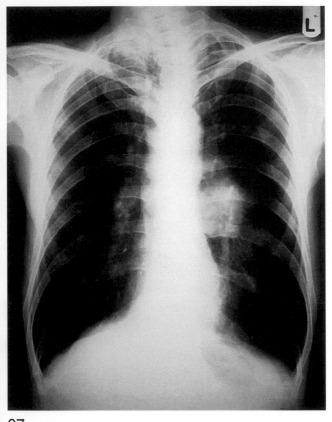

97. The photograph shows the chest X-ray of a patient who presented with painless dysphonia (hoarseness).

a. What is the abnormality shown on the X-ray?
b. What is the mechanism of the dysphonia?
c. What treatment options are available to improve this patient's voice?

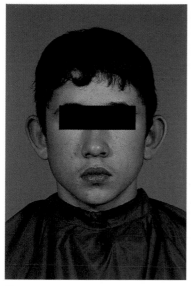

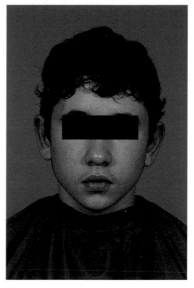

A   B

98. **This patient was distressed about the appearance of his ears and he was fed up being referred to as 'dumbo'! Photograph A is the pre-operative and photograph B is the post-operative appearance.**

a. Describe the abnormality.
b. What operation is used to correct this abnormality?
c. What is the main deformity giving rise to this appearance?

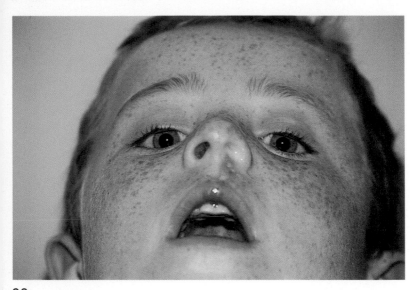

99. **The parents of this child brought him to the clinic because of foul smelling, unilateral nasal discharge of 3 weeks' duration.**

a. Describe the findings shown on the photograph and decide on the most likely diagnosis.
b. How is this condition managed?

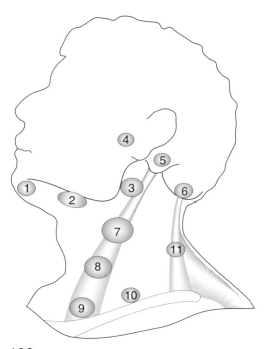

100. The diagram shows the various lymph node groups of the head and neck.

a. Name the groups shown 1–11.

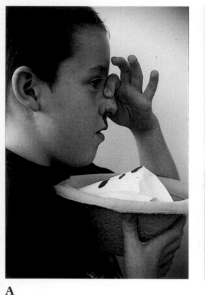 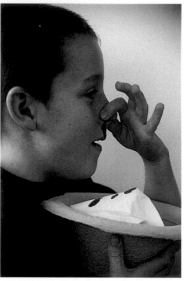

A   **B**

101. **The photographs show a patient being treated for a minor epistaxis (nose bleed).**

a. One of the photographs shows an incorrect technique. Which one is it?
b. Where do most nose bleeds come from?
c. Discuss the management of epistaxis.

Answers—Otology and Audiology

1.
   a. Pinna.
   b. External auditory canal.
   c. Middle ear space.
   d. Eustachian tube.
   e. Ossicular chain, composed of the malleus, incus and stapes.
   f. Vestibular labyrinth including the semi-circular canals.
   g. The cochlea.
   h. Internal auditory canal for the seventh (facial) and eighth (cochleo-vestibular) cranial nerves.

2.
   a. Pars tensa, which is often incorrectly called the tympanic membrane. The tympanic membrane also includes (b).
   b. Pars flaccida in the attic of the external auditory canal.
   c. The handle of the malleus. This is often used to help identify the position of the pars tensa.

3.
   a. The glossopharyngeal or ninth (IX) cranial nerve.
   b. From the diagram, it can be seen that sensory branches of the glossopharyngeal nerve supply the lining of the middle ear, the oropharynx and the base of the tongue. Some patients with oropharyngeal conditions, such as inflammation or tumour, get pain 'referred' to the ear. Hence patients with otalgia should have the oropharynx examined for pathology as well as the ear. An alternative cause for otalgia, that does not originate in the ear, is cervical osteo-arthritis.

4.
   a. Pure tone audiometry is best carried out in a sound-proofed booth. The patient wears a headset through which pure tones (usually at 250, 500, 1000, 2000, 4000 and 8000 Hz) are presented to each ear, in turn, at different sound levels (dBHL). The patient is told to indicate, usually by pressing a button, when they hear a tone. The quietest sound level at which a tone is heard is the air-conduction threshold at that frequency. These thresholds are marked on a chart: X for the left ear and O for the right ear. The procedure is then repeated, with masking as appropriate, with a bone-conduction vibrator placed on the mastoid behind each ear. This gives the bone-conduction thresholds shown as] for the left ear and [for the right ear.

b. The air-conduction thresholds indicate the degree of hearing impairment in each ear, the upper level of normal being an average over 500, 1000, 2000 and 4000 Hz of 25 dBHL. A pure-tone audiogram also indicates what type of hearing impairment there is. In a sensorineural impairment, the bone-conduction thresholds are the same as the air-conduction thresholds. In a conductive impairment, there is an air–bone gap, that is the bone-conduction thresholds are better than the air-conduction thresholds.

c. This patient has a mild sensorineural hearing impairment in the left ear and a severe conductive impairment in the right ear. (More accurately because the bone-conduction thresholds in the right ear are poorer than 25 dBHL, the patient has both a sensorineural and a conductive impairment, i.e. a mixed impairment in the right ear.)

5. Otitis media with effusion. Tympanometry is a technique in which an ear probe is sealed in the external auditory canal so that the pressure in the external auditory canal can be varied. A sound is then played into the ear canal, which is then reflected back and recorded by a microphone. The pressure at which most sound is reflected back is the middle ear pressure. In a normal tympanogram, the peak in pressure is between −100 and +200 mm H_2O. In otitis media with effusion, because there is fluid in the middle ear there is no peak in the graph, as is the case in the second tympanogram.

6. a. The patient's ability to keep their balance is being tested.

b. Keeping one's balance depends on the higher neurological pathways satisfactorily coordinating input from the proprioceptors in the limbs, from the vestibular labyrinth and from vision. In this test, vision has been eliminated by shutting the eyes. Abnormalities of the proprioceptors in the legs are extremely uncommon and are usually evident before doing the test by there being problems in walking. Hence, the Unterberger test is primarily a screening test of the vestibular labyrinth. If there is an uncompensated fault in the vestibular system, the patient will be unable to march on the spot in this manner without falling, moving about or opening their eyes.

7. Never. Commercially made cotton buds are of a size that are more likely to shove wax into the canal than to remove it. Normally, wax is shed spontaneously by epithelial migration along with the skin of the canal. Cleaning of normal external auditory canals is thus not only unnecessary but can be harmful.

8.
a. This child has a poorly developed pinna. The apparent opening is not the external ear canal but a blind pit. The ear canal is atretic. Hence hearing is the main concern. Cosmesis is only a secondary concern.

b. The child is aided initially with a bone-conduction hearing aid. When the child is older, this may be attached to a titanium peg which is screwed transcutaneously to the skull. Such pegs can also be used to attach prosthetic ears.

c. Clinically obvious congenital ear abnormalities are uncommon. Congenital sensorineural hearing impairments affect 2 children per 1000 live births and, in almost all of them, there is no external abnormality. Such children are best identified by neonatal screening of the hearing and are best managed with conventional hearing aids or, if profound, by a cochlear implant.

9.
a. This is an auricular haematoma, most likely caused by trauma to the cartilage, with secondary haemorrhage and a resultant collection of blood between the cartilage and the skin.

b. This requires to be aspirated with a syringe and a large bore needle. Thereafter, a pressure dressing should be applied for 24–48 hours to prevent the haematoma reforming.

c. The haematoma would absorb spontaneously but is likely to be associated with thickening of the cartilage and subcutaneous tissue resulting in a 'cauliflower ear'.

10.
a. This is an endaural incision (A). It is used to widen the external auditory canal to give better access to the middle ear. This approach is that most often used for surgery to improve the hearing by myringoplasty (repair of a perforation of the tympanic membrane), ossiculoplasty (reconstruction of the ossicular chain) or stapedotomy (replacing the stapes in otosclerosis).

b. This is a post-auricular incision (B). It lies over the mastoid, so gives easy access to the mastoid air cells to remove disease such as in active chronic otitis media (see Question 33). Access to the middle ear structures can also be obtained via this approach.

11.
a. It is likely to be either otitis externa or active chronic otitis media. Sometimes it can be both.

b. The ear requires to be cleaned of all pus and debris to allow otoscopy to be performed and to aid in management. The pus and debris can either be syringed or mopped out with cotton buds. Syringing is likely to be more effective in the hands of non-specialists and is not contra-indicated, even though there could be a perforation.

12. The normal external auditory canal has a bend in its cartilaginous outer third. This has to be straightened by pulling the pinna back and slightly up so that the speculum of an otoscope can be inserted to view the canal and tympanic membrane, usually by looking slightly anteriorly.

13.
a. The canal skin is swollen and inflamed. Though it could be a furuncle (boil), the most likely diagnosis is otitis externa.
b. The management is analgesics along with a topical ear preparation including steroids. Because the canal is oedematous, this is best applied as an ointment on a gauze wick which is changed daily until the canal opens up and topical steroid drops can then be used thereafter.

14.
a. Wax (cerumen) is blocking the view of the tympanic membrane.
b. It requires to be removed to visualise the tympanic membrane. This is best done by syringing.
c. It is unlikely to be the cause of the hearing impairment as the wax is not impacted. This is surmised because the wax is still in the outer third of the canal where it originates and a space can be seen between the wax and the canal.

15.
a. The canal skin postero-superiorly and the vessels over the handle of the malleus are hyperaemic. This is fairly frequent after uncomplicated syringing and should not cause concern. In this patient, the tympanic membrane is normal.
b. If properly carried out, syringing is unlikely to cause damage apart from hyperaemia of the skin of the canal. If roughly inserted, the syringe tip can traumatise the canal. If the water used for syringing is not at body temperature, the patient may have vertigo due to a caloric response. Traumatic perforations of the pars tensa do not occur due to the force of the syringed water. They can of course occur if the probe is inserted too far into the canal.

16. This cotton bud has been wound round a thin wire. A wooden orange stick would do just as well. The result is a thin bud with a fluffy end which can be used to clean the external auditory canal of pus and debris. This is most commonly required in active chronic otitis media and otitis externa. The mopping relieves the symptoms of discharge and smell as well as allowing topical medication to be delivered to where they are effective, i.e. through the perforation in active chronic otitis media and to the canal skin in otitis externa.

17.
a. There is a white bead, coated with wax in the canal.
b. The bead should be syringed out.
c. The bead has obviously been put in the canal by the boy himself. This is usually not done for fun but because the ear is sore and the boy was trying to relieve the discomfort. Hence, after syringing, other conditions such as acute otitis media, or negative middle ear pressure should be looked for.

18.
a. The patient has otitis externa. This is a dermatitis of the skin of the external auditory canal, in this instance provoked by a hot climate, swimming and perhaps self-poking the ear to relieve the discomfort.
b. The management is primarily aural toilet by syringing to remove the debris. The majority will settle with this management alone. Topical steroids without antibiotics will lessen the discomfort.

19.
a. The patient has an overgrowth of fungii (*Aspergillus niger*) on the canal skin. This is easily removed by syringing and the ear drops, certainly those which include topical antibiotics, should be stopped.
b. The antibiotics included in topical steroid ear drops are those not generally used systemically because of their side-effects, including oto-toxicity and nephro-toxicity. Gentamycin and Neomycin are those most commonly included. Their inclusion, along with topical steroids, is necessary for the effective management of active chronic otitis media (but not of otitis externa) and potentially can cause inner ear drainage, with vertigo and a sensorineural hearing impairment, if they come in contact with the round window membrane when there is a perforation. Fortunately, when the ear is active and the mucosa is inflamed, such complications are rare. However, topical antibiotics should always be stopped when the activity resolves in chronic otitis media.

20.
a. This is a 'red' tympanic membrane with increased vasculature over the handle of the malleus and round the periphery of the tympanic membrane. There are many potential reasons for this. It can occur in any fevered child. It can be a result of forceful otoscopy or it could be early acute otitis media.
b. Having ensured that there is no other cause for the fever, such as a urinary or upper respiratory infection, adequate hydration and analgesics such as Calpol are all that is required.

21.
a. Acute otitis media. The eardrum is generally inflamed and bulging as the ear is full of pus.
b. The initial management is of the fever, including adequate

hydration and of the pain with analgesics such as Calpol. In the majority, spontaneous resolution occurs within 24–48 hours without rupture of the pars tensa. In the majority of children, antibiotics have no role to play with acute otitis media.

c. The child should be seen about 48 hours later to ensure resolution has occurred. In about 5–10%, it will not have and it is these children that should be treated with antibiotics, usually Amoxycillin to prevent the rare development of mastoiditis or meningitis. All children should be seen 10–12 weeks later to ensure that otitis media with effusion has not resulted.

22.
a. The diagnosis is otitis media with effusion. The pars tensa is indrawn as is evident by the angle of the handle of the malleus. The indrawing is because of negative middle ear pressure as well as surface tension of the middle ear fluid. The pars tensa is yellowish in appearance due to the middle ear fluid. The pars flaccida is also retracted.

b. The diagnosis can be confirmed by tympanometry (Question 5). The child's hearing can be informally tested by free-field voice tests or better still by audiometry.

c. The main concern is the child's hearing rather than the pathology. Usually both will resolve with time. The parents are reassured that this is the case. Unfortunately, to date, no medication has been shown to hasten resolution. The child can be given an Otovent balloon to auto-inflate their ears (Question 24). Should the condition persist otoscopically after 10–12 weeks, the child should be referred for a more formal assessment of their hearing.

23.
a. The diagnosis is otitis media with effusion. The tympanic membrane is slightly indrawn as evident from the angle of the handle of the malleus and its colour is bluish due to the middle ear fluid. In a child of this age, the history of otalgia would suggest recurrent episodes of acute otitis media. Following these, the infection but not the fluid has resolved.

b. Some might argue that Amoxycillin has a role to play in encouraging resolution. However, the main concern is the hearing. Referral for this to be assessed is necessary and is relatively easily and reliably done in a child of this age by visual-reinforced audiometry.

24.
a. Blowing up a balloon via his nose. A commercial product 'Otovent' provides a plastic nose piece, along with some balloons, which makes this easier to do.

b. To auto-inflate his ears. Blowing up a balloon via the nose and with the mouth shut, increases the pressure in the nasopharynx. This usually opens up the Eustachian tube and forces air into the middle ear. There are two main reasons why someone might want to do this. The first is when there is a pressure differential between the middle ear and the external environment, such as following an aeroplane descent. The other is when there is otitis media with effusion (see Questions 22 and 23).

c. Yes. With instruction, most children over the age of 4 years can learn to auto-inflate their ears by this method. Hence, it is often prescribed to hasten resolution of childhood otitis media with effusion.

d. Valsalva technique.

25.
a. A ventilating tube (grommet), which in this instance is of blue plastic, has been inserted through a surgical incision in the pars tensa.

b. A ventilating tube allows air into the middle ear from the external auditory canal thus replacing the Eustachian tube which normally does this. Once the negative middle ear pressure has been relieved, the middle ear fluid drains down the Eustachian tube.

c. The natural history is for the ventilating tube to be extruded about 6 months later, by which time the otitis media with effusion will have resolved in the majority of children.

26.
a. A ventilation tube (grommet) has been inserted, most likely to improve the hearing in otitis media with effusion.

b. An infection has occurred around the ventilation tube. This occurs in about one-third of cases and is primarily because the ventilation tube is a foreign body and the child may be prone to recurrent episodes of acute otitis media. There is no evidence that getting water in the ear or going swimming increases the likelihood of infection.

c. The majority will settle with aural toilet (mopping or syringing) and topical antibiotics/steroid ear drops. If persistent, the ventilation tube can be remove.

d. In about 5% of ears that have had a ventilation tube inserted, the tympanic membrane will not heal spontaneously when the tube is extruded. A small permanent perforation results and this is thought more likely when there have been recurrent infections around the tube.

27.
a. This ear has two white plaques of tympanosclerosis, one anteriorly, the other posteriorly. These are areas of scarring and thickening of the fibrous tissue layer of the tympanic membrane. Inferiorly, there is a healed perforation that is

thinner than the rest of the eardrum and slightly retracted. The diagnosis is healed otitis media.

b. It is likely that this patient had acute otitis media, and/or otitis media with effusion, as a child. The healed perforation may also have been the site of a grommet, inserted to manage the otitis media with effusion.

c. The natural history is for the ear to stay the same. There may be a minor hearing impairment because of the scarring. No management is required.

28.

a. The diagnosis is inactive chronic otitis media. Posteriorly, there is a 60% permanent perforation of the pars tensa and there is a patch of white tympanosclerosis anteriorly. Through the perforation, the middle ear mucosa can be seen to be non-inflamed and there is no evidence of pus or inflammation. Hence the ear is inactive.

b. The preferred management is surgery. The eardrum can be repaired by a myringoplasty and, if the ossicular chain is disrupted as appears likely in this ear, the ossicular chain can be reconstructed by an ossiculoplasty. The combined operation is called a tympanoplasty. The alternative management is with a hearing aid but this requires servicing, is only effective when used, and may encourage the ear to become active.

29.

a. The diagnosis is active chronic otitis media. The ear is inflamed and there is some pus in the external auditory canal. This is not too obvious in the photograph as it had to be mopped out with a cotton bud to get a better view. The inflammation is primarily of the middle ear mucosa. This can be seen through a perforation of the pars tensa which is virtually total in extent. The white structures are the handle of the malleus anteriorly on the left and the stapes posteriorly on the right.

b. The management is initially of the activity with mopping and the installation of antibiotic steroid drops. The patient should be referred for surgical repair of the tympanic membrane—a myringoplasty. This will have the dual effect of preventing further episodes of activity and improving the hearing. In this particular ear, an ossiculoplasty is also required to improve the hearing as the stapes is no longer connected to the remainder of the ossicular chain because the long process of the incus has been eroded.

30.

a. The inexperienced might think that there is a perforation of the tympanic membrane posteriorly, i.e. on the left of the photograph. This is not the case. The eardrum is present but severely retracted and draped over the incus and stapes. In a perforation, the middle ear mucosa can be seen through the perforation as pink and slightly moist. This is not the case here.

b. The boy is likely to have had recurrent otitis media with effusion (glue ear) in the past.

c. The management is controversial but most physicians would be inactive and await events. Most likely nothing will occur but, in some, the retraction pocket could enlarge and the ear become active because squamous debris is retained in the pocket—a cholesteatoma. In others, the ossicular chain may be eroded and the hearing become worse. Some might advocate surgery but the condition is likely to recur despite this. Certainly the lad should be encouraged to auto-inflate his ear, either by doing a Valsalva manoeuvre or by using a nasal balloon (see Question 24). This will, hopefully, prevent further retraction.

31.
a. There is a crust of pus in the attic over the pars flaccida. The inexperienced might think this is wax.

b. The crust should be removed by syringing to see what lies below. Question 32 shows what lies below. The patient should be referred for a specialist otolaryngological opinion.

32.
a. In the attic, i.e. pars flaccida, there is an area of inflammation around some white debris. This debris is squamous epithelium in a skin-lined retraction pocket—a cholesteatoma. This is a variant of active chronic otitis media.

b. This patient has imbalance because the lateral semicircular canal of the vestibular labyrinth has been eroded by the inflammation.

c. The ear requires to be operated upon to remove the disease.

33.
a. The patient has had an open mastoid cavity created.

b. This would have been done for active chronic otitis media with a cholesteatoma, such as is shown in Question 32. The line drawings explain what was done. In A, the clinical appearance of the cholesteatoma is shown. In B, its relation to the underlying mastoid air cell system is shown. In C, the posterior bony canal wall has been surgically taken down to expose the disease in the mastoid which is then removed. This leaves an open mastoid cavity which heals with a lining of skin.

34.
a. If used for prolonged periods at full volume, this may damage your hearing.

b. Prolonged exposure to noise may cause a sensorineural hearing impairment. Some individuals are more susceptible to damage than others but, in general, the exposure has to equate to 8 hours a day over several years for this to occur. Exceptions to this are extremely loud sounds, e.g. in front of a professional loudspeaker in a club or explosives such as gunfire. Percussion power tools and motorcycling are also potentially damaging. Damage can be avoided by the correct wearing of ear defenders (Question 38).

35. The O-T-M switch is the O (off), T (telecoil) and M (microphone) on control. The telecoil is for use with an induction loop, for example in a telephone (see Question 36). The circular, knurled wheel controls the volume.

36. It indicates the availability of an induction loop, most frequently in a telephone but also in public places, such as churches, cinemas and theatres. A speaker's voice can be heard, with the exclusion of background noise, by induction if the listener is wearing a hearing aid set at the T (telecoil) position.

37. This is a noise generator or masker. It is worn by individuals with troublesome tinnitus. The open mould allows them to hear normally, but the noise of the instrument 'retrains' their central auditory system to disregard external noise and hence adjust to their tinnitus. Sometimes this instrument is used to mask out the tinnitus by being at a volume that the tinnitus is less obvious.

38. Ear defenders should be worn to protect the hearing whenever there is potential exposure to loud noise. They are most often used by those in noisy occupations, that is where it is difficult to communicate with fellow workers at a normal conversational distance without shouting or coming close to the listener's ear.

Answers—General Otorhinolaryngology

39.
a. This is a submandibular salivary gland calculus. This particularly large stone is shown protruding from the duct orifice in the anterior floor of mouth.
b. The calculus must be removed to unblock the duct. If the stone is in the body of the gland, excision of the submandibular gland itself may be required. In this case, the stone was excised from the duct, under local anaesthetic.
c. Calculi are commoner in the submandibular salivary gland because of the high mucin content of submandibular gland saliva.
d. Blockage of the duct with a stone leads to stasis and eventual abscess formation. More commonly, the prolonged stasis leads to duct stenosis and gland atrophy.

40.
a. There are symmetrically enlarged and inflamed tonsils which are touching in the midline. The features are those of tonsillitis.
b. In addition to clinical examination, a throat swab, a full blood count and glandular fever slide test may help in diagnosis.
c. The most likely diagnosis given the history (malaise, adenitis, failure to respond to antibiotics) is tonsillitis secondary to infectious mononucleosis (glandular fever).
d. As can be seen from the clinical photograph, tonsillar hypertrophy has reduced the airway in the oropharyngeal isthmus. Snoring is caused by vibration of soft tissues as air travels through a narrowing. Once the swelling has receded or the tonsils have been removed, the snoring is likely to improve.

41.
a. The picture shows severe bruising in the postauricular region extending down into the upper neck. This is often referred to a 'Battle's sign' and is associated with a fracture of the temporal bone and mastoid cortex.
b. The most likely diagnosis given the history and the clinical findings is a temporal bone fracture.
c. The patient is unable to walk without assistance because she is suffering from acute, severe vertigo as a result of damage to the inner ear sustained in the temporal bone fracture. After a variable period of time, the vertigo will settle as the patient

compensates by relying on the normal, contralateral
labyrinth.

d. A temporal bone fracture can be confirmed by CT scan views
of the skull base. Given her history of vertigo and tinnitus,
an audiogram would be essential to document the level of
hearing impairment sustained following the injury. In the
initial 24–48 hours following the trauma, the patient requires
neurological observation as she could develop an intra-
cranial haematoma with signs of increased intra-cranial
pressure.

42.

a. The picture shows bilateral periorbital bruising (black eyes),
a deformity of the external nose consisting of bruising over
the left nasal bone, depression of the left nasal bone and a
C-shaped external deformity.

b. The most likely cause of nasal obstruction in this patient is
a septal fracture-dislocation causing narrowing of one or
both of her nostrils. There is likely to be associated reactive
swelling of the nasal mucous membrane. A septal haematoma
which is a post-traumatic collection of blood in the
subperichondrial plane of the nasal septum must be
excluded. Clinically it is recognisable as a symmetrical
'boggy' swelling of the septum.

c. The most likely cause of numbness in her left cheek is
neuropraxia of the left infraorbital nerve.

d. First of all, ensure that she does not have a septal
haematoma. Nasal fracture manipulation within two weeks
of the injury, may correct the external appearance of the
nose. Septal deformities do not respond to nasal fracture
manipulation and require a septoplasty or septorhinoplasty, if
a cosmetic deformity persists.

43.

a. This neck lump is in the upper part of the anterior triangle
of the neck. The differential diagnosis includes
lymphadenopathy (benign and malignant), lesions of the
submandibular salivary gland, lesions of the lower pole of the
parotid gland, branchial cyst, aneurysm of the carotid artery
and carotid body tumour.

b. Photograph B shows fine needle aspiration being performed
to obtain tissue for cytology.

c. The photograph clearly shows the lesion to lie deep to the
anterior border of the sternomastoid and, if you look closely,
you can see turbid fluid in the hub of the needle and syringe.
Given that the lesion appears to contain turbid fluid, the
most likely diagnosis, taking all things into account, (position,
fluid content) is a branchial cyst.

d. All patients with a neck swelling should undergo a full

examination of the upper aerodigestive tract to exclude a primary lesion of infection or neoplasm in the oral cavity, nasopharynx, oropharynx, larynx or hypopharynx.

44.
a. This patient has multiple telangiectasias of the mucosal surface of his lower lip.

b. The patient is suffering from hereditary haemorrhagic telangiectasia (HHT or Rendu–Osler–Weber disease). This is an inherited autosomal dominant condition.

c. Iron deficiency anaemia in HHT is seldom due to the epistaxis. HHT patients have multiple telangiectasias of the mucosal surfaces of the gastrointrosternal tract and chronic undiagnosed gastrointestinal blood loss is a more likely cause of the iron deficiency anaemia.

d. There are multiple treatment options for the epistaxis. If the bleeding point can be found then it can be cauterised by using chemical (silver nitrate) or electro-cautery. Laser surgery has been used to cauterise small bleeding points and the application of skin grafts to the nasal mucous membrane has also been advocated to prevent the fragile telangiectases rupturing. Very often, however, prophylactic manoeuvres in this condition are unsuccessful and each bleeding vessel has to be dealt with individually.

45.
a. This endoscopic photograph shows a severe septal deviation. The septum can be seen to be touching the lateral nasal wall with the middle turbinate squashed in between.

b. The vast majority of septal deformities are of unknown aetiology, perhaps being developmental. Some are due to septal fractures following trauma.

c. The treatment for a severe septal deviation is a septoplasty. In the operation of septoplasty, mucosal flaps are elevated and the deviated part of the quadrilateral cartilage is resected and reshaped and the septum is repositioned in the midline.

46.
a. This is a contrast swallow radiograph more commonly referred to as a barium swallow. It clearly shows a large cystic dilatation with an air fluid level in the lower pharynx and upper oesophagus. This is the characteristic appearance of a pharyngeal pouch.

b. The pharyngeal pouch causes dysphagia by compressing the adjacent normal oesophagus and as a result of cricopharyngeal muscle spasm. Spasm of the circopharyngeus muscle (upper oesophageal sphincter) is thought to be important in causing the pouch to form.

c. Pharyngeal pouches fill with undigested foodstuff which stagnates and partially digests. This partially digested debris spills into the upper airway when the patient is recumbent and it is likely that this caused his aspiration pneumonia.

d. There are a number of ways of treating pharyngeal pouches. These can be summarised as open or closed techniques. The open approach involves a neck incision to isolate the pouch which is then excised and a cricopharyngeal myotomy is carried out to prevent recurrence of the pouch. Closed or endoscopic techniques divide the partition between the pouch and the normal oesophagus (in effect draining the pouch into the oesophagus). Closed techniques can be carried out using a laser or a stapling device and are often referred to as Dohlman's operation.

47.
a. This child has a hearing aid and a de-pigmented area of hair referred to as a white forelock.

b. The association of a white forelock, heterochromia of the iris and congenital sensorineural hearing loss is characteristic of Waardenburg's syndrome.

c. Waardenburg's syndrome is autosomal dominant in its transmission an is an example of a small number of rare, congenital syndromes which give rise to sensorineural hearing loss.

48.
a. Lesions in this area present with dysphonia (hoarseness).

b. The differential diagnosis of dysphonia includes lesions on the vocal cord (benign and malignant) abnormalities of cord mobility (vocal cord palsy), inflammatory lesions of the vocal cord (acute and chronic laryngitis) and functional (non-organic) disorders of voice production. It is important that all cases of dysphonia are considered to be due to laryngeal malignancy until proved otherwise.

c. This cyst at the anterior end of the left true vocal cord should be treated surgically using a special laryngeal endoscope and microscope to gain access. The cyst should be removed without damaging the normal anatomy of the vocal cord. Following such surgery, speech therapy may promote recovery.

49.
a. The picture shows a large ulcerative destructive lesion of the right temple and pinna region.

b. Differential diagnosis includes squamous cell carcinoma of skin, basal cell carcinoma, malignant melanoma and infective, inflammatory and vasculitic ulceration. This is a squamous cell carcinoma of the skin of the temple and pinna.

c. The geographical information is significant for two reasons: (1) The patient worked in Australia and exposure to strong sunlight over many years is thought to be important in the causation of squamous cell carcinoma of skin and (2) the patient's geographical isolation in the Australian outback may explain his late presentation with advanced disease.

d. Treatment options for squamous carcinoma of the skin include surgery (excision and reconstruction) radiotherapy or combined surgery and radiotherapy for advanced cases.

50.

a. This swelling is in the submandibular region and, therefore, the differential diagnosis includes lesions of the submandibular salivary gland, lesions of the lower pole of the superficial lobe of the parotid gland, lymphadenopathy (primary, secondary, benign or malignant). Lesions associated with the skin such as sebaceous cysts and lipomas. This was in fact a lipoma.

b. The investigation of choice is fine needle cytology which will provide diagnostic cytological information in over 90% of cases.

c. This is a trick question. Incisional biopsy is never recommended in this site. This is because of the disastrous consequences of incising either a pleomorphic adenoma or a squamous cell carcinoma (implantation of tumour into skin and adjacent tissue) and also because of the risk of damaging branches of the facial nerve in this region. Therefore, fine needle cytology should be carried out as the first line of investigation and, if in doubt, all lesions in this area should be referred to an otorhinolaryngologist.

51.

a. The photograph shows the middle turbinate and adjacent lateral nasal wall. Between these structures pus can be seen. The pus is coming from the middle nasal meatus which is the principle drainage pathway of the major sinus groups.

b. The diagnosis is subacute (3 weeks) purulent sinusitis.

c. Investigation and management of this case includes obtaining a sample of pus for bacteriology (nasal swab) and treating the patient with a nasal decongestant and an appropriate broad-spectrum antibiotic. If the patient fails to respond to this management, further investigation should not be carried out in a primary care situation and referral to an otolaryngologist is mandatory. Remember, pus under pressure in the sinus cavities is the second commonest cause of intracranial sepsis. Plain sinus X-rays do not provide any additional information and are known to be an unreliable investigation for sinusitis.

52.

a. The investigation is a contrast enhanced MRI scan of the brain and cerebellopontine angle regions.

b. The obvious abnormality is a rounded tumour in the right

cerebellopontine angle. This is characteristic of an acoustic neuroma.

c. The first-line investigation in a patient with unilateral tinnitus and hearing impairment is a pure-tone audiogram.

53.

a. The photograph shows the right nasal vestibule being held open with a nasal speculum. There is a papiliferous lesion filling the nasal cavity.

b. The differential diagnosis includes viral papilloma, inverted papilloma and carcinoma. Metaplastic nasal polyp or haemangiopericytoma are other rare possibilities. This is a viral papilloma.

c. Human papillomavirus.

54.

a. The differential diagnosis includes lymphadenopathy (primary, secondary, benign or malignant) lesions of salivary gland, thyroid gland, skin or adnexal structure (sebaceous cyst lipoma etc.), vascular lesions (aneurysm), carotid body tumour (haemangioma). The midline position makes a thyroglossal cyst the most likely diagnosis.

b. Photograph B demonstrates elevation of the cyst on tongue protrusion. This is due to connection of the thyroglossal cyst via a thyroglossal tract to the foramen caecum of the tongue.

c. Thyroglossal cysts should be excised in continuity with the middle portion of the hyoid bone (Sistrunk's operation). Failure to excise the middle portion of the hyoid increases the risk of recurrence.

55.

a. The photographs show a patient with severe right-sided facial swelling, erythema over the right maxilla, swelling around the right orbit and blood stained nasal discharge from the right nostril.

b. The most likely diagnosis is right-sided ethmoid sinusitis with orbital cellulitis as a complication.

c. This is an otorhinolaryngological emergency which requires specialist management. The principles of management are to secure drainage of the pus and to treat the infection. The patient will require surgical drainage of the maxillary antrum, frontal and ethmoid sinuses and high-dose broad-spectrum parenteral antibiotics.

d. Other complications of sinusitis include orbital abscess, meningitis, intracerebral abscess (frequently frontal lobe abscess), septicaemia, septic shock, cavernous sinus thrombosis, cerebral thrombophlebitis.

56.

a. The photographs show multiple ulcerative lesions, inflammation and sloughing of the hard and soft palate, and dorsum of the tongue.

b. The differential diagnosis of aggressive oral ulceration includes herpetic gingivostomatitis, apthous ulceration, mucosal candidiasis, vasculitic ulcers, Beçhet's disease, systemic lupus erythematosis.

c. This is herpetic gingivostomatitis and this can be confirmed by viral swab and culture and raised serological titres to herpes virus.

d. The management of this patient relies on rehydration and correction of any electrolyte imbalance. Intravenous fluids, adequate analgesia in the form of surface anaesthetic, e.g. benzocaine lozenges, use of virocidal and antiseptic mouthwashes, e.g. Povidone-iodine mouthwash. There is debate over the efficacy of Acyclivor once the ulceration has reached this stage, but it is the author's belief that it accelerates resolution and reduces morbidity.

57.
a. This is a subconjunctival haemorrhage and the two types are: (1) with a posterior limit and (2) without a posterior limit. From what we can see in the photograph, this does not appear to have a posterior limit. The absence of a posterior limit is seen in cases of skull base fracture.

b. Subconjunctival haemorrhages are a non-specific indicator of trauma to the eye. In the absence of eye trauma, however, it can signify an anterior skull base fracture. This is also suggested by the absence of a posterior limit to the subconjunctival haemorrhage.

c. It is very difficult to decide whether unilateral watery rhinorrhoea is CSF or not and, therefore, any patients with this sign should be referred for a specialist opinion. In the past, detection of elevated glucose levels in the fluid was thought to be a useful test but this has now been superseded by the detection of beta-transferrin in the fluid.

58.
a. The most likely cause of this appearance is a carcinoma.

b. The diagnosis can be established by incisional biopsy which can be carried out under local anaesthetic in the clinic. (It is, however, important to obtain a representative sample, by avoiding any areas of necrotic tissue.)

c. It is very important to examine the oral cavity in detail, in particular, noting any fixation of the lesion to the mandible. Examination of the remainder of the upper aerodigestive tract paying particular attention to the mucosal surfaces of the mouth, pharynx and hypopharynx is also mandatory. The neck should be examined for evidence of metastatic lymphadenopathy. Mucosal carcinomas of the upper aerodigestive tract can be multiple.

59.
a. This is the skin-prick test in which dilute quantities of allergen are injected intradermally and the presence or absence of an allergic response recorded. The test allows the causal allergens to be identified in patients with allergic rhinitis. The bottles of reagent each contain a solution of a single allergen.

b. Anaphylactic shock is a rare but most significant risk of carrying out this test and, therefore, it should only be carried out where resuscitation equipment is immediately available. The management of anaphylactic shock includes securing the airway, lying the patient flat, elevating the feet in order to improve venous return and administration of intramuscular adrenalin (0.5–1 ml of 1:1000 solution). In addition to this, the patient should be given oxygen and intravenous chlorphaniramine 10 mg and 100 mg of hydrocortisone. Intravenous access should be established and intravenous fluids commenced and, if the patient deteriorates, assisted ventilation may be required.

60.
a. Differential diagnosis includes squamous cell carcinoma, basal cell carcinoma, vasculitic ulcer, chondrodermatitis nodularis helicis and traumatic ulcer. This is a squamous cell carcinoma of the pinna.

b. Diagnosis can be confirmed by an excision biopsy, although sometimes fine-needle cytology can provide the answer.

c. Treatment options include surgical excision, radiotherapy or a combination of both. A lesion such as the one shown could be excised and the defect reconstructed using a local rotation flap or a full thickness skin graft.

d. Examination of the lymph node drainage tracts of the head and neck is mandatory to check for metastatic spread.

61.
a. The features are those of a left lower motor neurone facial palsy.

b. Idiopathic (Bell's palsy). Trauma including surgery (e.g. middle ear surgery, parotid surgery, temporal bone fracture). Middle ear disease (cholesteatoma, chronic otitis media). Herpes oticus (Ramsay–Hunt syndrome), malignant parotid neoplasms, HIV infection, sarcoidosis, Melkersson–Rosenthal syndrome (recurrent facial palsy in patients with deeply furrowed tongues).

c. The most important thing in idiopathic facial palsy is to protect the eye. Inability to close the eye properly leads to corneal drying and ulceration. The patient should apply ointment to the eye and wear an eye pad at night. The role of steroids in idiopathic facial palsy is controversial and, in the majority of cases, of no advantage. Therefore, eye cover and

reassurance is usually all that is required in an idiopathic
nerve palsy.

62.
a. The clinical photograph shows diffuse symmetrical
enlargement of the anterior lower part of the patient's neck.
The MRI scan reveals this to be due to a large homogenous
thyroid swelling consistent with a large goitre. The differential
diagnosis is simple colloid goitre, thyrotoxicosis, Hashimoto's
disease, thyroiditis, thyroid carcinoma.
b. Definitive cytological diagnosis can often be achieved by fine-
needle aspiration cytology.
c. The presence of hoarseness is a worrying symptom and is
suggestive of a thyroid malignancy invading the recurrent
laryngeal nerve.

63.
a. There is a rounded swelling lying posterior to the posterior
border of the sternomastoid, i.e. in the posterior triangle of
the neck. There is no overlying erythema and the lesion
appears to be solitary.
b. Differential diagnosis of any neck lump includes
lymphadenopathy (inflammatory or neoplastic: primary,
secondary, benign or malignant), lesions of the skin and
subcutaneous tissues, (e.g. a sebaceous cyst, lipoma), vascular
abnormalities, (e.g. aneurysm), congenital abnormalities, (e.g.
branchial cyst, thyroglossal cyst).
c. As with all neck swellings, a detailed history and full clinical
examination can often suggest the diagnosis. Examination of
the upper aerodigestive tract may also give a clue to the
nature of the lesion, but fine-needle aspiration cytology is
probably the most reliable investigation. This turned out to be
a tuberculous gland. Mycobacterial infection has a
predilection for the nodes in the posterior triangle.
d. If this node is to be excised, (e.g. if cytology did not provide
the answer), the surgeon should be aware of the proximity of
the accessory nerve (cranial nerve eleven) in the floor of the
posterior triangle.

64.
a. The photograph clearly shows paralysis of the left side of
the tongue with the tongue deviated to the affected side.
This is characteristic of a hypoglossal nerve palsy (cranial
nerve 12).
b. Looking closely at the photograph, we can see the tip of a
white plastic prosthesis in the midline of the patient's neck.
This is a voice rehabilitation prosthesis, thus the patient has
undergone a laryngectomy for laryngeal cancer. Therefore,
the most likely cause is direct invasion of the hypoglossal
nerve by laryngeal cancer.

65.
a. The pictures show a red, swollen mass in the left submandibular region and a carious lower left molar. The diagnosis, therefore, is submandibular lymphadenopathy with abscess formation secondary to dental sepsis.
b. This condition needs a two-pronged approach. Firstly, incision and drainage of the abscess with antibiotic cover and, secondly, dental treatment to remove the source of the infection.
c. Dental infections are frequently due to the streptococcus but often by the time an abscess is established, there is a mixed population of both aerobes and anaerobes, therefore, an antistreptococcal (penicillin) antibiotic is required and, in addition, Metronidazole is used to deal with the anaerobes.

66.
a. The right nostril clearly shows broadening of the columella with the skin of the columella touching the nasal ala. On the left, the pink of the nasal septum is clearly visible obstructing the nostril. Therefore, this is a dislocation of the inferior end of the nasal septum into the right nostril with a corresponding bend of the septum to the left posteriorly.
b. Severe septal deviation.
c. Most septal deviations are idiopathic although many are a result of trauma.
d. The treatment involves a septoplasty which aims to centralise the septum.

67.
a. Lacrimal sac mucocele (swollen lacrimal sac containing infective secretions as a result of a blocked lacrimal drainage system), Arcus Senilis.
b. The most likely diagnosis is nasolacrimal duct obstruction.
c. Treatment for nasolacrimal duct obstruction involves drainage of the lacrimal sac via a surgically created opening into the nasal cavity. Otolaryngologists are increasingly involved in this type of surgery because of the high level precision which can be achieved in endoscopic nasal surgery. The operation is called dacrocystorhinostomy.

68.
a. From the picture it can be seen that the patient has an irregular scar running across the middle of the neck. There is absence of the laryngeal prominence and the most striking feature is a tracheostomy with a white plastic object in the 12 o'clock position. Therefore, the patient has had a total laryngectomy which is carried out almost exclusively for laryngeal carcinoma.
b. The white structure visible in the photograph is a Blom Singer voice prosthesis. This is a one-way valve which fits between the tracheostomy and the reconstructed pharynx.

Using the valve, the patient can shunt air into the pharynx and obtain a reasonable voice using the walls of the pharynx to produce sound which is then modified by the resonators of the oral cavity and the articulators of the tongue, teeth and lips.

c. The alternatives to tracheo-oesophageal prosthesis for speech rehabilitation include: (1) oesophageal speech in which the patient learns to swallow air and then regurgitate it. This produces a characteristic explosive burping type of speech; (2) use of an electro-mechanical device to produce sound waves in the oral cavity by vibrating the tissues of the floor of mouth; and (3) least favourable are non-verbal means of communication.

69.
a. This is a large parotid tumour and the most common lesion in this area is a pleomorphic salivary adenoma.

b. As with most lumps in the head and neck, fine-needle cytology is the first investigation to be carried out. The important point is that these lesions should not be biopsied because of the risk of seeding and damage to the facial nerve.

c. The operation of choice is a superficial parotidectomy in which the lesion is removed with a surrounding area of normal parotid gland taking care to preserve all of the branches of the facial nerve. Simple excision or enucleation of these lesions is associated with high incidence of implantation and recurrent disease and should, therefore, not be carried out.

70.
a. This is a lateral soft tissue X-ray of neck which shows considerable widening of the tissues behind the larynx in the prevertebral plane.

b. The most likely diagnosis in this case is a post-cricoid carcinoma.

c. Investigations must include endoscopy of the region which is best carried out using rigid endoscopes. In addition, a full blood count and nutritional assessment should be undertaken.

d. As with all malignancies in the head and neck, treatment options are surgery, radiotherapy or combinations of both. Surgery for this lesion would necessitate a pharyngolaryngoesophagectomy and reconstruction using either interposed stomach or a free jejunal graft. Radical radiotherapy may be more applicable in a patient of this age.

71.
a. The photograph shows a perforation of the anterior part of the nasal septum.

b. The septal perforation may be caused by trauma such as surgery, nasal injury or nose picking! It may also be due to inflammatory conditions including Wegener's granulomatosis, sarcoidosis, tuberculosis, syphilis. Rarely, a malignant tumour can destroy the septum.

c. It is very difficult to close nasal septal perforations although a number of surgical operations have been described. In some patients, the perforation can be plugged using a special plastic obturator. Most patients, however, are successfully managed using a simple ointment to prevent the crusting and drying out associated with the turbulent airflow around the perforation.

72.
a. The slide shows marked swelling of the anterior neck and loss of the normal contours. There is an area of ulceration in the midline of the neck.

b. The most likely cause of swelling and skin breakdown is an advanced carcinoma of the larynx or pharynx. This patient had advanced laryngeal cancer which had involved the strap muscles and skin of the neck.

c. Management of head and neck cancer involves surgery, radiotherapy and combinations of both. This advanced cancer will necessitate total laryngectomy, excision of the involved skin and reconstruction prior to radical radiotherapy.

73.
a. In all tongue ulcers, the possibility of a carcinoma should be top of the list. Other causes of ulceration are vasculitic ulcers, infective ulcers, traumatic ulcers, syphilis and aphthous ulceration.

b. Investigation should involve a history, full examination of the upper aerodigestive tract, examination of the neck and biopsy of the lesion.

c. The anterior part of the tongue has bilateral drainage, therefore, lymph nodes in the left submental and submandibular region may drain the right side of the tip of the tongue and vice versa.

74.
a. The patient has a grossly deformed nose. The nasal bones deviate to the patient's right with a concavity in the region of the left nasal bone. The nasal tip is displaced to the patient's left giving an overall C-shaped deformity.

b. This type of deformity is most often caused by a punch or blow from the patient's left hand side. For example, the deformities are likely to have been produced by a punch from a right-handed assailant.

c. The operation of septorhinoplasty allows correction of the external bony and cartilaginous deformities and straightening of the septum to improve both the cosmetic and functional defects.

75.
a. The slide shows an area of skin occupying the lateral part of the oropharynx in the region of the tonsillar fossa and the adjacent soft palate. This is the appearance of a cutaneous flap reconstruction following excision of an oropharyngeal cancer. The commonest donor sites are a pectoralis major myocutaneous flap or free radial forearm skin flap.

b. Following major oropharyngeal resections, patients have problems with swallowing and will often require nutritional support for a period of time. Speech is also affected due to difficulty with articulation caused by impaired mobility of the tongue. Loss of oropharyngeal sensation can often lead to aspiration and choking when eating. The operation can often be disfiguring and patients will require psychological support and counselling in some instances.

c. Patients who have had cancer of the upper aerodigestive tract are at an increased risk of developing a second primary cancer, especially in the lung. Second primary bronchial cancers are a frequent cause of death in patients who have had successful treatment of a head and neck tumour.

76.
a. The CT scan shows complete bony obstruction of the right posterior nares. This is a unilateral choanal atresia.

b. Choanal atresia is usually diagnosed in the neonatal or early infant period when the nasal obstruction causes problems with feeding. Bilateral choanal atresia can cause neonatal respiratory distress but unilateral choanal atresia as in this case may often go unnoticed.

c. The patient complains of total nasal obstruction on the right side and the airway can be improved by opening up the bony plate using perforators or special nasal drills.

77.
a. Squamous cell carcinoma, basal cell carcinoma, malignant melanoma, kerato-acanthoma.

b. Surgery, radiotherapy or laser therapy could all be used to remove this lesion depending on the diagnosis. This is a squamous cell carcinoma and surgery was chosen in order to ensure complete excision of the lesion.

c. Once the lesion has been surgically excised, there will be a large defect on the nasal tip. This can be closed by rotating adjacent skin, for example from the nasolabial fold in a local rotation flap, or as was used in this case, by using a full thickness skin graft from the post-auricular region.

78.
a. This is a vocal cord haematoma involving the anterior end of the right true vocal cord. It is a result of haemorrhage into the cord caused by very loud shouting.

b. Conservative management would include voice rest in the

hope that the haematoma will gradually organise and resolve. If this does not occur then microlaryngeal endoscopic surgical excision is indicated.

c. Strict voice rest is required or, better still, changing the football team he supports!

79.

a. There is severe swelling of the left pinna with an unhealed laceration occupying the conchal region. The bruising and swelling in the region of the concha has obliterated the normal contours of the pinna. He has an auricular haematoma which has become infected giving rise to infection of the cartilage known as perichondritis.

b. This complication may have been prevented by ensuring evacuation of all blood clot at the time of the original presentation and application of a pressure bandage.

c. The condition now requires formal incision and drainage, debridement of the wound edges, application of a pressure bandage and use of high-dose broad-spectrum antibiotics.

80.

a. The tube shown in photograph A has a cuff. The function of the cuff is to provide a seal around the tube to enable positive pressure ventilation and to prevent secretions, or blood etc., tracking down the trachea into the lung.

b. A non-cuffed, plastic tracheostomy tube may be used in patients who require regular tracheobronchial suction but have a competent larynx which will prevent aspiration around the tube.

c. Long-term tracheostomy patients require supplementary humidification to moisten the air which is bypassing the nose and going straight to the lungs. It is also important to provide a means for the patient to communicate; this can be done either in the form of a speaking valve or a fenestrated tube for patients who still have a larynx. Blockage of a tracheostomy tube with secretions would be a potentially disastrous circumstance and, therefore, patients should either be taught how to change and clean their tracheostomy tube themselves or this should be carried out by nursing staff.

81.

a. The anterior triangle is delineated superiorly by the mandible, laterally by the anterior border of the sternomastoid, and has its apex inferiorly in the manubrial notch. The posterior triangle is bounded anteriorly by the posterior border of sternomastoid, inferiorly by the clavicle and posteriorly by the anterior border of trapezius. The apex of the posterior triangle lies superiorly in the region of the occiput.

b. The lesions are situated in the posterior triangle.

c. The lesions are most likely to be lymph nodes which may be secondary to infection in the scalp, tuberculosis, metastasis from head and neck carcinoma, lymphoma, thyroid carcinoma, breast or apical lung lesions.

d. Investigations should involve a complete head and neck examination, chest X-ray, examination of the breasts and fine-needle cytology of the lesions. Serological investigations should include a full blood count, glandular fever slide test and ESR.

82.

a. Basal cell carcinoma, squamous cell carcinoma, actinic keratosis, malignant melanoma.

b. These are basal cell carcinomas and the management consists of local excision ensuring complete removal of the tumour.

c. Elderly, wrinkled skin is ideally suited for hiding incisions and tends to produce flat, cosmetically acceptable scars. The lesions are close to the nasolabial crease and this would allow excision and primary closure with minimal cosmetic deformity.

83.

a. The photograph shows swelling in the region of the right parotid gland and herpes labialis on the lower lip.

b. The patient has become debilitated and dehydrated leading to acute bacterial parotitis. Herpes labialis is an indication of a generally stressed immune system.

c. Acute parotitis should be treated by a high fluid intake, good oral hygiene, intravenous rehydration as required, broad-spectrum antibiotics and analgesia. Failure to resolve may lead to parotid abscess formation. Herpes labialis is usually self-limiting and by the time vesicles have appeared, acyclovir is not indicated. In this patient, application of povidone-iodine would help reduce viral shedding, and spontaneous resolution is likely to occur as his general condition improves.

84.

a. This is a maxillectomy specimen which contains the maxilla, and the floor and contents of the right orbit. The operation is, therefore, an extended total maxillectomy and orbital clearance.

b. Total maxillectomy and orbital clearance is indicated for advanced tumours of the maxillary sinus which by the time of diagnosis have extended to involve the lateral nasal wall, ethmoid sinuses, floor of the orbit and orbital contents.

c. Paranasal sinus malignancy usually presents late. Small tumours within the maxillary antrum are largely asymptomatic. Therefore, tumours only present when they have invaded adjacent structures such as the nasal cavity (epistaxis, nasal obstruction, unilateral nasal polyp), orbital

contents (proptosis, diplopia, infra-orbital nerve dysaesthesia)
or skin of the face (ulceration).

85.
a. This patient has a severe saddle deformity with collapse of
the supratip region of the nose. The nasal bones are intact
and, therefore, this is a cartilaginous saddle.
b. Cartilage destruction can be produced by trauma, septal
haematoma, surgical resection, neoplasia, sarcoidosis,
tuberculosis, Wegener's granulomatosis, syphilis or idiopathic.
c. The combination of nasal cartilage destruction and renal
failure suggests the diagnosis of Wegener's granulomatosis
which is a multi-system granulomatous inflammation
involving the respiratory tract, nasal mucosa and kidneys.
Blood should be taken for a C'ANCA estimation.

86.
a. Squamous cell carcinoma of the tongue.
b. Biopsy of the margin of the tumour.
c. Full examination of the mouth, pharynx and neck to evaluate
spread of the disease to adjacent structures such as mandible,
floor of mouth, buccal mucosa. Examination of the upper
aerodigestive tract for simultaneous lesions elsewhere and for
evidence of lymph node metastasis. This type of examination
often takes place under anaesthetic, as a so-called staging
examination.
d. As with all squamous cell carcinomas of the head and neck,
surgery, radiotherapy and combinations of both form the
mainstay of treatment. Depending on the stage of the
tumour, either radical radiotherapy or radical excision and
reconstruction are indicated.

87.
a. This is most likely to be a frontal sinus mucocele which is a
collection of inflammatory fluid within a blocked frontal
sinus. As it gradually enlarges, it erodes adjacent bone.
b. After a full ENT examination, paying particular attention to
the nose and sinuses, the patient should undergo nasal
endoscopy and coronal CT scanning of the paranasal sinuses.
c. The frontal sinus can be approached endonasally via an
endoscopic approach or externally by incisions placed in the
eyebrow or a bi-coronal incision placed behind the hairline
allowing the skin overlying the frontal bone to be turned
inferiorly as a flap. A mucocele of this size would almost
certainly require an external approach.

88.
a. The photograph shows both vocal cords. An area of white,
irregular tissue occupies most of the right true vocal cord
with a similar area affecting the middle portion of the medial
border of the left true cord. The right side is most involved
but there also appears to be a problem on the left side.

b. Dysphonia (hoarseness) is the most likely presenting symptom.

c. The most likely diagnosis is squamous cell carcinoma of the vocal cord. As with all tumours of the head and neck, this can be treated by radiotherapy, surgery or combinations of both depending on the stage of the tumour. In early tumours, radical radiotherapy can produce cure rates in excess of 90% whilst in the more advanced disease, total laryngectomy and follow-up radiotherapy is required thus emphasising the importance of early diagnosis.

89.

a. The contrast radiograph shows a sharp, shelf-like, filling defect in the upper oesophagus. This is the appearance of an oesophageal web.

b. Given the history and the X-ray appearance, this is characteristic of Brown Kelly–Paterson's syndrome also known as Plummer–Vinson syndrome.

c. The syndrome of oesophageal web, iron deficiency anaemia, atrophic gastritis and koilonychia is associated with a significantly elevated risk of post-cricoid and cervical oesophageal carcinoma.

90.

a. The patient has a cutaneous abscess overlying the left nasal bone.

b. This is the so-called 'danger area' of the face because venous drainage from this area passes to the intracranial circulation via the cavernous sinus.

c. As with all abscesses, the principle of surgical drainage and antibiotic treatment should be applied. This particular condition should be treated aggressively in order to avoid the risk of cavernous sinus thrombosis, meningitis or cerebral thrombophlebitis.

91.

a. This is a coronal CT scan of the nose and paranasal sinuses.

b. It shows a large opacification in the right maxillary antrum. This is consistent with a cyst or polyp in the right maxillary antrum.

c. Access can be gained either endoscopically via the nose making an opening in the lateral nasal wall, referred to as an antrostomy. Alternatively, a sublabial incision would allow us to gain access to the anterior wall of the maxilla which can be opened via a sublabial antrostomy.

92.

a. Indirect laryngoscopy using a headlight and an angled mirror is the standard way to examine the larynx. This is gradually being replaced by fibreoptic per-nasal endoscopy of the larynx which can also be carried out in the outpatient clinic.

b. Leukoplakia.

   c. The differential diagnosis includes dysplasia (mild, moderate, severe), carcinoma in situ, squamous cell carcinoma.

93.
   a. This is a unilateral nasal polyp.
   b. Unilateral nasal polyps require specialist investigation including nasal endoscopy, examination of the nasopharynx and CT scanning of the nose and paranasal sinuses. Only when a full examination of the nasopharynx and scanning has been carried out can excision or biopsy be contemplated.
   c. A unilateral nasal polyp could in fact be an encephalocoele, meningocoele, angifibroma, transitional cell papilloma, olfactory neuroblastoma, carcinoma or lymphoma.

94.
   a. The photograph shows swelling in the right lower neck overlying the thyroid gland.
   b. Full head and neck examination, paying close attention to the mouth, pharynx and larynx, should be followed up with fine-needle aspiration cytology, and ultrasound of the lesion.
   c. Unilateral swelling of the thyroid associated with dysphonia raises the possibility of a thyroid malignancy causing invasion of the recurrent laryngeal nerve, therefore, indirect laryngoscopy is mandatory in such a patient.

95.
   a. The photograph shows a puncture wound overlying the upper part of the neck on the left. The X-ray confirms a radio-dense foreign body lying within the structures of the neck at a level deep to the skin entry wound. Close inspection of the outline of the foreign body shows the characteristic appearance of an airgun pellet.
   b. Penetrating neck injuries may damage vascular structures (internal jugular vein, external jugular vein, carotid artery), neurological structures (facial nerve, sensory nerves, hypoglossal nerve, accessory nerve etc.), bony structures (cervical spine, mandible, skull) visceral structures such as larynx and pharynx.
   c. As with all penetrating neck injuries, the principles of ABC (Airway, Breathing and Circulation) apply. (A) ensure that there is an adequate and secure airway; (B) that the patient is breathing and not in need of respiratory support and (C) that the patient's circulatory system is adequate, i.e. the patient has not entered hypovolaemic shock. Care must be taken to secure haemostasis and also rule out any related trauma to adjacent structures. Once the patient is stabilised, the foreign body can be removed but this will require an experienced surgeon and full operating facilities.

96.
   a. This is a squamous carcinoma until proved otherwise.
   b. Whilst the aetiology of squamous cell carcinoma of the oral

cavity is unknown, there are strong associations with smoking, chewing tobacco, alcohol consumption and, in some parts of the world, chewing betel nut.

c. As with all squamous cancer of the head and neck, treatment options include surgery, radiotherapy and combinations of both. Chemotherapy is often used as an adjuvant treatment but its value is debatable.

97.

a. The X-ray shows a large opacity in the left hilar region. This is characteristic of a bronchial carcinoma.

b. The most likely cause of hoarseness is involvement of the left recurrent laryngeal nerve by tumour in the hilum or metastatic mediastinal nodes (remember the left recurrent laryngeal nerve descends into the chest before looping around the arch of the aorta).

c. Most patients with unilateral vocal cord palsy will achieve some degree of compensation with time as the contralateral normal cord adapts to the new position of the paralysed cord. However, if dysphonia persists and is troublesome, various cord medialisation techniques can be used. These include injecting teflon lateral to the paralysed vocal cord to move it medially or the same can be achieved by an external operation which places a silicone wedge lateral to the vocal cord.

98.

a. In photograph A, the patient can be seen to have bilateral prominent ears. This is often incorrectly referred to as bat ear deformity.

b. The operation of pinnaplasty or otoplasty is used to correct the deformity and it relies on creating new folds and bends in the cartilage of the pinna to reduce the lateral projection of the ears. It can be seen in photograph B that this has produced a reasonable cosmetic improvement.

c. The principal deformity is a developmental lack of the antihelix. The aim of the pinnaplasty operation is to create a new antihelix.

99.

a. The photograph shows unilateral, left-sided purulent rhinorrhoea which is associated with redness and inflammation around the nasal vestibule (vestibulitis). Unilateral nasal discharge in a child should be considered due to an impacted foreign body until proved otherwise.

b. Gentle suction removal of the pus in the outpatient clinic should allow examination of the anterior part of the nose where the foreign body may be visible. Foam-rubber, vegetable matter (peas etc.) or silver foil are among the more common foreign bodies seen. Often the patient will require a general anaesthetic in order to remove the foreign body. It is important not to try to remove the foreign body without access to full otorhinolaryngology support as inadequate lighting and instrumentation will often lead to the child being hurt and a total loss of confidence. Therefore, if in doubt, refer to otorhinolaryngology. Once the foreign body has been removed, the inflammation usually settles, but use of an antibiotic ointment such as mupirocin is a worthwhile addition to treat the vestibulitis.

100.
1. Submental nodes.
2. Submandibular nodes.
3. Jugulo-digastric nodes or tonsillar nodes.
4. Pre-auricular or parotid nodes.
5. Post-auricular or mastoid nodes.
6. Occipital nodes.
7. Upper deep cervical nodes.
8. Mid deep cervical nodes.
9. Lower deep cervical nodes and para-tracheal nodes.
10. Supra-clavicular nodes.
11. Posterior triangle nodes.

101.
a. Photograph A shows an incorrect technique. Pressure is being applied over the nasal bones and this will achieve nothing. The correct technique is shown in photograph B where the alar region has been compressed against the lower anterior part of the nasal septum. This is the correct way to apply the so-called Hippocratic technique for control of epistaxis.
b. Most nose bleeds come from Little's area in the anterior inferior part of the nasal septum. This is why pressure to the alar regions will stop the majority of nose bleeds.
c. The management of epistaxis depends on the type and severity of the bleeding. Bearing in mind ABC (for Airway Breathing and Circulation), we should ensure that the patient is adequately resuscitated and then attempt should be made to identify the source of the bleeding. The nose is examined using a headlight, nasal speculae and suction. If the bleeding point can be found, it can be cauterised using either chemical (silver nitrate) or electro-cautery. Failure to find the bleeding point should initiate a search with a nasal endoscope which is obviously a specialised technique. In the Accident and Emergency Department, it may be necessary to insert gauze packing or special balloons into the nose to try to control the bleeding. Bleeding of a severity to necessitate nasal packing should be referred immediately to an Otorhinolaryngologist.

Suggested Reading

Browning, G. G. *Clinical Otology and Audiology*,
2nd Edn. Butterworth Heinemann, Oxford, 1998
ISBN 0 7560 3373 5

Coleman, B. H. *Diseases of the Nose, Throat and Ear, and Head and Neck*,
14th Edn. Churchill Livingstone, Edinburgh, 1992
ISBN 0 443 04563

Becker, W., Naumann, H. H., Pfaltz, C. R. Edited by Buckingham, R. A.
  Ear, Nose and Throat Diseases—A Pocket Reference,
2nd edn. Thieme Verlag, New York, 1994
ISBN 313 671 2021

Browning, G. G. *Updated ENT*,
3rd Edn. Butterworth Heinemann, Oxford, 1994
ISBN 0 7506 1921 X

Wormald, P. J., Browning, G. G. *Otoscopy—A Structured Approach*
Arnold, London, 1996
ISBN 0 340 613769

- Question 2—Fig 2.7a
- Question 13—Fig. 3.17
- Question 14—Fig. 9.12a
- Question 15—Fig. 8.2
- Question 17—Fig. 6.2
- Question 18—Fig. 6.9
- Question 19—Fig. 6.12
- Question 20—Fig. 6.3
- Question 21—Fig. 6.5
- Question 22—Fig. 5.3
- Question 23—Fig. 5.8
- Question 25—Fig. 4.19
- Question 26—Fig. 5.13
- Question 27—Fig. 4.21
- Question 28—Fig. 4.8
- Question 29—Fig. 3.12
- Question 30—Fig. 8.6
- Question 31—Fig. 7.30
- Question 32—Fig. 7.7
- Question 33—Fig. 7.38

Index

Note: entries are indexed **by question numbers** and matching answers.

Abscess over nasal bone, 90
Acoustic canal, *see* Auditory canal
Acoustic neuroma, 52
Adenoma, pleomorphic salivary, 69
Allergic rhinitis, 59
Anaphylactic shock, skin-prick test, 59
Antibiotics, ototoxicity, 19
Aspergillus niger, 19
Audiometry, pure tone, 4
Auditory canal
    external, 1
        inflammation, *see* Otitis externa
        otoscopy and the cartilaginous part of, 12
        surgical widening, 10
    foreign body, 17
    internal, 1
Auditory ossicles, *see* Ossicular chain
Auricle, *see* Pinna
Autoinflation of ears
    nasal balloon, 24, 30
    Valsalva manoeuvre, 24, 30

Bacterial infections, *see also specific pathogens*
    dental, 65
    parotid, 83
Balance problems, *see also* Vertigo
    cholesteatoma, 32
    Unterberger test, 6
Balloon, nasal, 24, 30
Basal cell carcinoma, 82
Bat ear, 98
Battle's sign, 41
Bleeding/haemorrhage
    nasal, *see* Epistaxis
    subconjunctival, 57
Blom Singer voice prosthesis, 68
Boil, 13
Branchial cyst, 43
Bronchial carcinoma, 97
Brown Kelly–Paterson syndrome, 89

Calculus, salivary, 39
Cancer (predominantly carcinoma)
    bronchial, 97
    laryngeal, *see* Laryngeal cancer
    oral, 58, 86, 96
    paranasal sinus, 84
    pharyngeal, 72, 75
    skin, 49, 60, 77, 82
    thyroid, 62, 94
    vocal cord, 88
Carcinoma, *see* Cancer
Cartilage
    external ear, otoscopy and, 12
    nasal, destruction, 85
Cellulitis, orbital, 55
Cerebellopontine angle tumour, 52
Cerumen, *see* Wax
Choanal atresia, unilateral, 76
Cholesteatoma, 32, 33
Cochlea, 1
Congenital ear disorders, 98

with sensorineural hearing impairment, 8, 47
Cotton buds, 16
    warning, 7
Cranial nerves, XIIth, palsy, 64
Cyst
    branchial, 43
    maxillary antrum, 91
    thyroglossal, 54
    vocal cord, 48

Deafness, *see* Hearing impairment
Dental infections, 65
Dysphonia (hoarseness)
    bronchial carcinoma, 97
    thyroid cancer, 62, 94
    vocal cord cyst, 48

Ear defenders, 38
Eardrum, *see* Tympanic membrane
Endaural incision, 10
Epistaxis
    management, 101
    Rendu–Osler–Weber syndrome, 44
Ethmoid sinusitis, 55
Eustachian tube, 1

Facial palsy, idiopathic, 61
Foreign body
    ear, 17
    neck tissue, 95
    nose, 99
Fracture
    nasal, 42
    old, 74
    temporal bone, 41
Frontal sinus mucocele, 87
Fungal infection, external ear, 19
Furuncle, 13

Gingivostomatitis, herpetic, 56
Glandular fever, 40
Glossopharyngeal nerve, 3
Glue ear, *see* Otitis media
Granulomatosis, Wegener's, 85
Grommets (ventilation tube), 25
    complications, 26

Haematoma
    pinna (auricle), 9, 79
    septal, 42
    vocal cord, 78
Haemorrhage, *see* Bleeding
Haemorrhagic telangiectasia, hereditary, 44
Hearing
    impairment
        in inactive chronic otitis media, management,
        28
        sensorineural, *see* Sensorineural hearing
        impairment
        wax and, 14
    protection, 38
Hearing aids, 8, 28

O-T-M control, 35
Hereditary haemorrhagic telangiectasia, 44
Herpes labialis, 83
Herpetic gingivostomatitis, 56
Hippocratic technique, epistaxis, 101
Hoarseness, see Dysphonia
HPV, 53
Human papillomavirus, 53
Hypoglossal nerve palsy, 64

Imbalance, see Balance problems
Induction loop and telephones, 35, 36
Infraorbital nerve, left, neuropraxia, 42
Injury, see Trauma
Inner ear trauma, 41

Labyrinth, vestibular, see Vestibular labyrinth
Lacrimal sac mucocele, 67
Laryngeal cancer (carcinoma), 72
  hypoglossal nerve invasion, 64
  post-cricoid, 70
  voice prosthesis, 68
Laryngeal nerves, recurrent
  bronchial cancer invading, 97
  thyroid cancer invading, 62, 94
Leukoplakia, vocal cord, 92
Lipoma, submandibular, 51
Lung carcinoma, 97
Lymph nodes (neck)
  draining tongue, 73
  location, 100
Lymphadenopathy (neck), 81
  submandibular, 65
  tuberculous, 63

Malignant tumours, see Cancer
Malleus, 2
Masker, tinnitus, 37
Mastoid cavity/air cells, surgical access, 10, 33
Maxillary sinus/antrum
  cancer, 84
  cyst or polyp, 91
Maxillectomy, 84
Middle ear, 1
  inflammation, see Otitis externa
Mononucleosis, infectious, 40
Mucocele
  frontal sinus, 87
  lacrimal sac, 67
Myringoplasty, 29

Nasal bones
  abscess overlying, 90
  trauma, 74
Nasal cavity
  papilliferous lesions, 53
  polyp, 93
Nasal septum, see Septum
Nasolacrimal duct obstruction, 67
Neck
  lumps/swellings
    differential diagnosis, 43, 62, 63, 81
    malignant, 62, 72, 94
    non-malignant, 43, 63, 83

  thyroid swelling, 62, 94
  nodes, see Lymph nodes; Lymphadenopathy
  penetrating injuries, 95
Neoplasms, see Tumours
Neuroma, acoustic, 52
Noise, hearing impairment, 34
Noise generator (tinnitus), 37

Obstruction
  nasal, causes, 42, 74
  nasolacrimal duct, 67
Oesophageal speech, 68
Oesophageal web, 89
Oral cancer, 58, 86, 96
Orbital cellulitis, 55
Orbital clearance, maxillary sinus advanced cancer,
  84
Oropharyngeal cancer, 75
Ossicular chain, 1
  reconstruction, 29
Otitis externa, 11, 13, 18
  cleaning pus/debris, 16
  steroid therapy, complication, 19
Otitis media
  acute, 21, 27
  chronic active, 11, 29
    antibiotic/steroid drops, 19
    with cholesteatoma, 32, 33
    cleaning pus/debris, 16
    surgical access, 10, 33
  chronic inactive, hearing impairment,
    management, 28
  with effusion (glue ear), 22, 23, 27
    autoinflation, 24
    grommets, see Grommets
  recurrent, 30
  tympanometry, 5
O-T-M control, 35
Otoplasty, prominent ears, 98
Otoscopy and the cartilaginous part of external
  auditory canal, 12
Outer ear, see Otitis externa and specific structures

Papilliferous lesions, nasal cavity, 53
Paranasal sinuses, see Sinuses; Sinusitis
Parotid
  bacterial infection, 83
  pleomorphic adenoma, 69
Pars flaccida, 2
  attic over
    inflammation, 31
    pus crust in, 31
Pars tensa, 2
Paterson–Kelly syndrome, 89
Penetrating injuries, neck, 95
Perichondritis, pinna, 79
Pharyngeal cancer, 72, 75
Pharyngeal pouch, 46
Pinna (auricle), 1
  congenital deformity, 8
  haematoma, 9, 79
  squamous cell carcinoma, 49, 60
  surgical incision behind (for mastoid cavity
    access), 10, 33

Pinnaplasty, prominent ears, 98
Pleomorphic salivary adenoma, 69
Plummer–Vinson syndrome, 89
Polyp (arising from paranasal sinus)
    maxillary antrum, 91
    in nasal cavity (= nasal polyp), 93
Post-auricular access to mastoid cavity, 10, 33
Pouch, pharyngeal, 46
Pulmonary carcinoma, 97
Pure-tone audiometry, 4

Rendu–Osler–Weber syndrome, 44
Rhinitis, allergic, 59
Rhinorrhoea, unilateral
    purulent, 99
    watery, 57
Rodent ulcer (basal cell carcinoma), 82

Saddle deformity, nose, 85
Salivary glands
    calculus, 39
    tumour, 69
Schwannoma, acoustic (acoustic neuroma), 52
Sensorineural hearing impairment
    congenital, 8, 47
    noise exposure, 34
    pure tone audiometry, 4
Septo(rhino)plasty, 45, 66, 74
Septum, nasal
    deformities/deviation, 45, 66, 74, 85
    haematoma, 42
    perforation, 71
Sialolithiasis, 39
Sinuses (paranasal)
    cancer, 84
    cyst, 91
    mucocele, 87
    polyp, see Polyp
Sinusitis
    ethmoid, 55
    subacute purulent, 51
Skin carcinoma
    basal cell, 82
    squamous cell, 49, 60, 77
Skin-prick test, 59
Squamous cell carcinoma
    oral, 58, 86, 96
    skin, 49, 60, 77
    vocal cord, 88
Stone, salivary, 39
Streptococcal dental infections, 65
Subconjunctival haemorrhage, 57
Submandibular gland, calculus, 39
Submandibular lymphadenopathy, 65
Submandibular region, swelling, 50
Surgery, ear, incisions, 10
    for mastoid cavity access, 10, 33
Syringing (ear), 14, 15
    foreign body, 17

Telangiectasia, hereditary haemorrhagic, 44
Telecoil, 35
Telephone induction loop, 35, 36
Temporal bone fracture, 41
Thyroglossal cyst, 54
Thyroid swelling, 62, 94
    malignant, 62, 94
Tinnitus, noise generator, 37
Tongue
    carcinoma, 58, 86, 96
    paralysis of left side, 64
    ulcer, 73
Tonsillitis, 40
Tracheo-oesophageal voice prosthesis, 68
Tracheostomy tube, 80
Trauma, see also Fracture
    ear
        external, 9, 79
        inner, 41
    nasal, 42, 74
    neck, penetrating, 95
Tuberculous lymph nodes, 63
Tumours
    benign
        cerebellopontine angle, 52
        salivary gland, 69
    malignant, see Cancer
Tympanic membrane (eardrum), 2
    flaccid part, see Pars flaccida
    otoscopy, 12
    'red'/inflamed, 20, 21
    severely retracted, 30
Tympanometry, otitis media with effusion, 5
Tympanoplasty, 28
Tympanosclerosis, 27

Ulcer
    rodent (basal cell carcinoma), 82
    tongue, 73
Unterberger test, 6

Valsalva manoeuvre, 24, 30
Ventilation tube, see Grommets
Vertigo, inner ear damage, 41
Vestibular labyrinth, 1
    screening test, 6
Vocal cord
    cancer, 88
    cyst, 48
    haematoma, 78
    leukoplakia, 92
    palsy, voice improvement, 97
Voice prosthesis, laryngeal cancer (carcinoma), 68

Waardenburg's syndrome, 47
Wax (cerumen), removing, 14
    warning, 7
Web, oesophageal, 89
Wegener's granulomatosis, 85